Basic Health Publications User's Guide to Propolis, Royal Jelly, Honey, and Bee Pollen

Learn How to Use "Bee Foods" to Enhance Your Health and Immunity.

C. Leigh Broadhurst, Ph.D.

Jack Challem Series Editor

The information contained in this book is based upon the research and personal and professional experiences of the author. It is not intended as a substitute for consulting with your physician or other healthcare provider. Any attempt to diagnose and treat an illness should be done under the direction of a healthcare professional.

The publisher does not advocate the use of any particular healthcare protocol but believes the information in this book should be available to the public. The publisher and author are not responsible for any adverse effects or consequences resulting from the use of the suggestions, preparations, or procedures discussed in this book. Should the reader have any questions concerning the appropriateness of any procedures or preparations mentioned, the author and the publisher strongly suggest consulting a professional healthcare advisor.

Series Editor: Jack Challem
Editor: Cheryl Hirsch
Typesetter: Gary A. Rosenberg
Series Cover Designer: Mike Stromberg
Basic Health Publications User's Guides are published by Basic Health Publications, Inc.
www.basichealthpub.com

ISBN: 978-1-59120-163-2 (Pbk.)
ISBN: 978-1-68162-870-7 (Pbk.)

CONTENTS

INTRODUCTION

The honeybee (*Apis mellifera*) is the world's most popular insect. Native to Europe, it has been introduced successfully in every continent except Antarctica. Bees thrive from Russia and Scandinavia through the Tropics and "down under" in Australia and New Zealand. The immense value of honeybees to the world is not commonly appreciated.

According to the U. S. Department of Agriculture, one mouthful in three of the foods you eat directly or indirectly depends on pollination by honeybees. Honeybee pollination is worth 14 billion dollars annually to the agriculture industry.

Apiculture is the formal name for commercial beekeeping. Apiculture was practiced in ancient Egypt, Mesopotamia, Greece, Rome, India, and China. Ancient Buddhist, Christian, Hindu, Moslem, and Native American cultures revered the honeybee, as do their modern counterparts. China has a 3,000-year continuous tradition of apiculture. In the 1600s, workers in Shenyang collected 2,500 to 3,000 kilograms of honey each year just to supply the Emperor's Palace.

Did you know that throughout history apiculture has been just as important for providing medicine as it has food? Beekeepers were usually among the longest-lived individuals in a town or village, due to their prodigious consumption and use of beehive products.

These valuable beehive products are honey, propolis, bee pollen, and royal jelly. In this book the many natural health uses of apiculture are brought up to date and scientifically documented. Let me give you an idea of how you and your family can benefit from these amazing substances:

- *Honey* is the world's best-known treatment for burns, infected wounds, and skin ulcers. It can kill wound bacteria that are resistant to antibiotic drugs. Using honey as a sweetener instead of sugar adds antioxidant protection to your diet.
- Taking *propolis* daily can reduce both the number of respiratory infections you contract during the winter season and their severity. Propolis salve is a highly effective treatment for herpes. It is also one of the most effective herbal detoxifiers and antioxidants known, and as such can benefit people with chronic diseases from arthritis to cancer.
- A teaspoon of *bee pollen* provides you with a quick and easy way to eat the equivalent of one large serving of vegetables. Bee pollen is an effective treatment for hay fever, prostatitis, and varicose veins.
- Taking *royal jelly* daily can reduce your risk for cardiovascular disease and strengthen your immunity. It's also a superior cosmetic ingredient for moisturizing and smoothing facial wrinkles.

Honey, propolis, bee pollen, and royal jelly each have their own chapter in this book that's more or less self-contained. However, it's important that you at least skim Chapter 1 first because many important terms are defined there that will be used throughout the book. This also makes Chapter 1 the most demanding to read in the book, but worth investing your time and attention.

Each chapter includes details from research studies that explain how bee products work medicinally. These sections are more scientific than others in the chapter and you do not need to read them to use this book.

Please take the time to understand this fascinating and truly helpful information about beehive products. The natural health uses of honey, propolis, bee pollen, and royal jelly are so diverse that *any* household can find something that applies. After you've read this book, I guarantee you will appreciate the honeybee as never before!

CHAPTER 1

Honey—Sweet Protection against Infection

Honey is made from flower nectar that is collected by worker honeybees in spring, summer, and early autumn. Some worker bees also collect "honeydew" from the sugary secretions of aphids that feed on tree sap. The nectar is greatly concentrated and is stored in wax cells, thousands of which form the honeycomb. In a natural honeybee colony, honey serves as food for the bees through the winter when plants are dormant. In an apiculture hive, where most of the honeycomb is removed to extract the honey and beeswax, the beekeeper provides the bees with sugar or a corn-syrup solution to sustain them.

Beekeepers earn most of their income by renting their bee colonies to farmers and orchardists. The hives are transported to the places where important crops are in bloom, and the bees "work for food," gathering nectar and pollen while pollinating the crops. Pollinating California's almond trees alone takes about 1 million bee colonies. Honey is the tasty result of all this pollination effort.

The Composition of Honey

For millennia, honey has been appreciated for its delicious sweet flavor and digestibility. Honey is 15 to 21 percent water by weight, and almost all of the remainder is carbohydrate. About 85 percent of the solids in honey are the simple sugars glucose and fructose. There are minor amounts of sucrose, maltose, and other sugars—the exact composition varies with the honey.

The sugar molecules in honey are strongly attracted to the water and bond to it. This is one reason why honey is a viscous syrup instead of a crystalline solid like table sugar (pure sucrose). If an attempt is made to dry out honey, it will rapidly reabsorb water from the atmosphere and return to its liquid state.

Honey does crystallize sometimes. Crystallization can happen spontaneously in a jar that has been on the shelf for a while, or honey can be purposely crystallized by the manufacturer to make spreadable honey products. However, crystalline honey is still sticky and contains lots of water; it is not dry and spoonable like pure sucrose crystals.

A few percent of honey consists of *phytochemicals* from the various nectar source plants. These phytochemicals cause endless variation among honeys, similar to the effects of adding various herbs, spices, or extracts to plain bread. Unprocessed or lightly processed honey always retains the flavor and aroma of the nectar source plants, and this is what *really* makes it special.

Phytochemicals
Natural, biologically active chemicals made by plants, such as lycopene in tomatoes and watermelon, quercetin in tea and onions, anthocyanins in grapes and bilberry, and menthol in spearmint and pennyroyal.

Raw, unprocessed honey is like fine wine—the source plants, growing location, season, climate, weather, processing, and just plain luck influence the color, aroma, and flavor. Commercial beehives may be placed in orange groves to produce fragrant orange-scented honey, or in white clover fields to produce light, mild, all-purpose clover honey. Buckwheat flowers produce strong, dark, musky honey that's an excellent substitute for molasses in baking or barbecue sauce. However, buckwheat honey like buckwheat pancakes is definitely an acquired taste for the gourmet palate!

Honey Is an Herbal Tonic

When the word "phytochemical" is used in the fields of nutrition and natural healing, it refers to the phytochemicals that people eat and use medicinally. These phytochemicals have measurable health effects on our metabolism. The various phytochemicals in honey not only influence taste and aroma, but they also provide antioxidant protection, healing properties, and nutritional benefits.

Luckily for us apicultural scientists are interested in identifying the phytochemical composition of honey for several reasons. Most important, the trace phytochemicals in honey provide scientists with a "fingerprint" that can be used to identify the source plants visited by the bees. The phytochemicals in honey can be extracted and then compared to phytochemical extracts from likely source plants near the hives where the honey originated.

In a given foraging area, there are potentially many source plants sampled in any type of honey produced. But in practice, bees visit favorite plants again and again, presumably because these plants provide more abundant and nutritious nectar and pollen.

Identifying preferred source plants is also important so that beekeepers know where to locate hives and what plants to grow to help keep bees healthy and productive. There are also some source plants that beekeepers don't want bees to visit: on occasion wild tropical honeys poison animals because the flowers of the source plants are poisonous to mammals but not to insects.

There's also a legal aspect to phytochemical fingerprinting. In order for honey to be labeled "unifloral," meaning from a single floral source, 51 percent of the nectar or 45 percent of the traces of pollen in the honey must be from the designated source plant. Although these percentages may seem low (can you imagine orange juice that's only required to be 51 percent from oranges?), there's no practical way to control bees more than this!

Over time, characteristic phytochemical patterns in popular honey varieties began to emerge, and it was not lost on the researchers that many of these "fingerprint" phytochemicals are biologically active ingredients in herbal teas and medicines. For example, Australian *Eucalyptus* sp. honeys are identified by small amounts of eucalyptus essential-oil components (linalool, 1,8 cineole, menthol, and others) and the *flavonoids* myricetin, luteolin, tricetin, and kaempferol. Orange honey has a small amount of orange essential oil (citral, limonene) and the flavonoid hesperetin. Likewise, honeys from sage, rosemary, thyme, and heather have small amounts of the respective essential oils, which result in distinctive aromas and flavors in the honeys and contribute medicinal benefits.

Flavonoids

A huge class of phytochemicals that are widely distributed in food and medicinal plants. The basic three-ring skeleton of all flavonoids consists of two phenol (hydroxybenzene) rings linked to a pyran ring.

Antioxidants in Honey

Floral honeys tend to have relatively high levels of phytochemicals that act as antioxidants. This is because the honey contains some of the antioxidants that the source plant manufactures. All living creatures create *reactive oxygen metabolites* (ROM), also called free radicals, as unavoidable byproducts of metabolism. Plants need antioxidant protection just like we do to keep ROM under control. Otherwise these free radicals damage tissues and cause inflammation. Degenerative arthritis is a good example of what happens to us when ROM are not controlled.

Reactive Oxygen Metabolites (ROM)
Also called free radicals, ROM are highly reactive, strongly oxidizing chemical compounds.

Immune system responses unavoidably produce ROM because limited amounts of reactive oxygen have value in killing pathogens and flushing tissues clear of toxic substances. ROM are also produced in immediate responses to trauma, such as car accidents, flesh wounds, falls, sports injuries, or broken bones. Among other actions, they prompt enzymes involved in damage control, clean up, and sterilization to begin their work. ROM cause acute (intense but of limited duration) inflammation, warmth, and swelling at the wound site. Of course, this can be painful, yet it is also beneficial because it sets the healing process in motion.

In chronic (ongoing) inflammatory conditions such as arthritis, tendonitis, asthma, and ulcers the inflammation process keeps going beyond what is wholly beneficial. For some reason, our bodies just can't quit while they're ahead! Chronic inflammatory conditions are characterized by an *excess* of ROM, which irritates tissues and interferes with healing instead of helping it.

Antioxidants act like chemical sacrificial lambs. They react more quickly and readily with ROM than our cells do. ROM are disabled when they react with the "sacrificial antioxidants" so they can't continue to irritate us.

Luckily, many of the antioxidant phytochemicals in plants work just as well for us! We gain antioxidant protection from eating fruits and vegetables and from using herbs—and also by using honey instead of refined sugars.

In laboratory studies, the antioxidant capacity

of nineteen samples of commercial, unifloral honey from fourteen plant sources was tested. The highest antioxidant content was found in Illinois buckwheat honey, and the lowest in California sage honey. Water tupelo, Hawaiian Christmas berry, sunflower, and buckwheat were the four honeys with the highest antioxidant content, although buckwheat stood alone at the top of the class. The buckwheat honey was twenty times richer in antioxidants than the sage!

Buckwheat honey was also tested on humans and found to increase their bloodstream antioxidant ability. In this study, twenty-five male subjects drank five different beverages: water, black tea, black tea with buckwheat honey, black tea with sugar syrup, or water with 80 grams of buckwheat honey. Although tea is known to be rich in antioxidant phenolics, tea with or without honey did not increase antioxidant ability—only honey with water did. It's thought that the phenolic antioxidant compounds in buckwheat honey were more easily absorbed than those from tea.

Four studies concur that the darker the color of the honey, the higher its antioxidant content. Common, lighter transparent honeys such as clover, orange, soybean, and mesquite were unremarkable in their antioxidant content. In contrast, buckwheat, water tupelo, and eucalyptus are dark-brown translucent honeys.

Phenolics

Phenolics consist of linked benzene rings to which with hydroxide (OH) groups are attached. Black tea tannins and grape seed extract are two common examples. All flavonoids are phenolics.

The major antioxidant phytochemicals in honey are identical to those that have already been identified in fruits, vegetables, and herbal products. Darker honeys are dark precisely because they contain higher concentrations of phenolics, which impart brown or dark-yellow colors. This higher phenolic content mostly accounts for the increased antioxidant activity. Vitamin C (ascorbic acid) and other organic acids such as malic, gluconic, and cinnamic are also important antioxidants in honey.

The major antioxidant flavonoids found in all temperate climate honeys studied are pinobanksin, pinocembrin, chrysin, and galangin. Honeys such as Hawaiian Christmas berry and neem contain different flavonoid and phenolic antioxidants because the source plants are tropical.

Compositional variation also occurs in Southern Hemisphere honeys such as Australian *Eucalyptus* sp. (red river gum, mallee, and yellow box, for example). Bees in this part of the world sample very different plants than those in Europe and North America, but this doesn't affect their ability to make honey and prosper.

Honey has a tremendously long shelf life compared to a sugar-water solution of similar concentration and viscosity. One reason is that its natural antioxidants and essential oils act as preservatives. Honey is a safe, natural preservative for foods such as sausage, deli meats, and precut produce.

Five percent honey (by weight) mixed into cooked ground turkey was more effective in preventing the oxidation of turkey fat during refrigerated storage than the food antioxidants BHT and vitamin E. The oxidation of fat during storage is what gives leftover meat a stale or rancid off-flavor. A dry honey rub was similarly effective for cooked or raw sliced turkey. Dipping fresh-cut fruits such as apples and pears into honey slows the appearance of browning from enzymatic oxidation. Soybean, buckwheat, and tupelo honeys are among the best choices for preservative honeys.

Making Honey Part of Your Healthy Diet

Using darker aromatic honeys daily instead of refined sugar or corn syrup is like adding an herbal tonic or an extra serving of produce to your diet, but it is not a substitute for fruits and vegetables. Overall, honey is lower in phytochemicals and much higher in sugar than fruits and vegetables, so it should *replace* refined carbohydrates in your diet. It should *not replace* fruits, vegetables, or herbal preparations. We can be *very* healthy from eating several pounds of produce each day, but several pounds of honey would not be recommended!

Most people use honey in tea or coffee, or on toast or pancakes. You can also make your own barbecue sauces, salad dressings, vegetable dips, and other condiments with honey instead of using commercial brands that contain sugar or corn syrup. It's a good idea to stir honey and one-eighth to one-quarter teaspoon vitamin C powder into fruit salad to keep it fresh longer and to improve its nutrition. With a little creativity honey can be a significant source of beneficial phytochemicals in your diet.

Heating and processing destroys the natural vitamin C and most of the organic acid antioxidants in raw honey. While it's great to use flavorful honey for cooking and baking, bear in mind some medicinal properties are lost.

Antibiotic and Antiseptic Uses of Honey

As mentioned earlier, honey was revered for its healing properties in the ancient world. Islamic, Greek, Roman, Chinese, Egyptian, Sub-Saharan African, and Native American cultures all used honey medicinally. Honey has been used for treating sore throats, colds, flu, skin and stomach ulcers, diarrhea, indigestion, and for dressing wounds. Recent research has confirmed the healing properties of honey. It is a broad-spectrum antibiotic, inhibiting the growth of numerous pathogenic bacteria, and an effective antifungal agent.

The incidence of antibiotic-resistant infections in hospitals and clinics has risen dramatically, to the point where some surgical patients must be quarantined. Most of these infections are caused from *Staphylococcus sp.* (staph) bacteria. If you have a large wound, surgical incision, or other type of septic wound, and the skin bacteria in the area cannot be controlled, then you're at tremendous risk for disfiguring scars, or even a life-threatening infection.

The noted honey researcher Dr. Peter Molan from the University of Waikato in New Zealand has studied the antimicrobial aspect of honey for years. In over thirty published articles, honey reportedly cleared up infections that were unresponsive to conventional antiseptics and antibiotics. Honey quickly healed wounds that were infected with dangerous strains of *Staphylococcus* that are resistant to penicillin or to multiple antibiotics.

Dr. Molan and his colleagues cultured *Staphylococcus aureus* and *Pseudomonas sp.* bacteria collected directly from the infected wounds of patients. These bacteria can cause gangrene if left unchecked. Dressings with any variety of raw honey prevented bacterial growth in the wounds, even when diluted seven to fourteenfold by body fluids. Normally, dressings are changed several times a day, so honey would never even become this diluted. Brazilian researchers have found tropical South American honeys to be similarly effective against *Staphylococcus aureus.*

Antimicrobial activity is generally greater in stronger-tasting honeys from aromatic plants such as mints, culinary herbs, conifers, sagebrushes, heathers, and barberries. And as with antioxidant activity, darker honeys tend to have greater antimicrobial activity than lighter honeys.

Manuka Magic

New Zealand's manuka honey is an example of a floral honey that is considered superior for medicinal use. The essential oil extracted from the manuka tree (*Leptospermum scoparium*) has long been used topically to prevent or cure fungal and bacterial infections; to soothe diaper rash, dermatitis, and psoriasis; and to kill oral bacteria in mouthwashes and rinses. The healing properties of the essential oil are shared by the dark, fragrant honey.

Psoriasis
An autoimmune disease in which skin cells are overproduced, resulting in scaly, flaky, dry skin that is easily irritated and may be very unsightly.

In the studies described above in which bacteria from infected patient wounds were cultured, maunka honey was the most effective out of the fifty-eight honeys tested against *Staphylococcus aureus* bacteria. Manuka honey could still kill *Staphylococcus* even when diluted to one part in fifty-six! Manuka honey was also far more effective than mixed pasture honey against *Pseudomonas sp.* bacteria.

Acids produced by oral bacteria are responsible for eroding dental enamel and eventually causing cavities. A chewable "honey leather" made with manuka honey was found to be twice as effective as sugarless gum in reducing plaque levels on teeth and gum bleeding. For three weeks, thirty participants chewed or sucked either the manuka-honey product or gum for ten minutes, three times a day, after each meal. The antibacterial effect of the manuka honey was so strong that it overrode the potentially detrimental effect of the honey sugars with respect to tooth decay.

Healing Wounds with Honey

Ancient warriors carried raw honey with them to treat battlefield wounds. It was known that cuts, abrasions, or burns covered with a layer of honey would heal more rapidly, with less chance of infection. Raw honey mixed with propolis was also utilized, as we will discuss in the next chapter.

According to a review by Dr. Molan, honey has been used successfully to heal many types of wounds and lingering or chronic skin infections. In interviews with more than 600 wound patients who used honey on wounds, no irritation, pain, allergy or other adverse reactions were reported. Honey is equally effective at healing large and small mammals recovering from veterinary surgery or experimentally induced wounds.

Here's a summary of honey's amazing wound-healing properties:

- Honey reduces infection, pain, inflammation, weeping (oozing), and foul odors.
- Honey dressings soothe the pain and itching of wounds, as well as soften scabs and gently debride crusts and dead tissue.
- Honey heals wounds faster and more cleanly than other treatments.
- Wounds treated with honey heal with less scarring and better tissue regeneration.
- Honey actively promotes the growth of healthy new skin.

In most cases, honey was called in to treat tough cases that weren't responding to conventional treatment. For example, modern medicine has no effective treatment for persistent mouth sores, a side effect of radiation treatment for cancer. Indonesian patients with head and neck cancer that had developed mouth sores were given 15 milliliters of honey before and after treatment with radiation. Honey reduced the severity and pain of the sores compared to standard care (nothing!). In addition, honey made it possible for 30 percent more patients to eat properly during radiation therapy.

Consider what a welcome relief the honey was for patients suffering from these tough cases.

Honey was also found to be the only treatment that healed diabetic ulcers, which had festered for one to three years. Honey debridement (removal of dead tissue) from sore, infected wounds was found to confer an enormous advantage over surgical debridement, which is an exceedingly painful process. There were also patients whose wounds were literally untouchable, and could not have their wounds properly cleaned until honey dressings were utilized.

Clinical Success Stories

Honey has been the subject of a wide variety of research experiments and has an impressive list of clinical trials compared to most natural products. Here are some highlights demonstrating its healing properties:

- In a 1991 clinical trial with burn patients, treatment with honey was evaluated against a control group, which received conventional treatment with gauze soaked in silver sulfadiazine (SS). After seven days, 91 percent of the honey-treated burns were free from infection compared to only 7 percent for the SS-treated burns. After fifteen days, 87 percent of the honey-treated wounds were healed versus 10 percent in the SS group. The honey had formed a flexible, protective barrier over the burn area, which prevented infection, absorbed pus, and reduced pain, irritation, and odors. In addition, the enzymes in honey appeared to stimulate the growth of new tissue.
- In two other 1993 and 1994 randomized clinical trials, gauze impregnated with honey healed burns faster than either polyurethane film (an average of 10.8 versus 15.3 days, respectively) or amniotic membrane (9.4 versus 17.5 days, respectively). Only 8 percent of forty patients treated with honey had residual scars compared to 17 percent of twenty-four patients

treated with amniotic membrane. Amniotic membrane is a very expensive and specialized wound dressing as compared to honey and gauze. Moreover, the honey-treated burns were free from infection in seven days.

- British surgeon and burn specialist Dr. Subrahmanyam, who performed the studies above, has also reported the successful storage of skin grafts in honey at room temperature. There was a 100 percent success rate for the graft uptake after six weeks storage, and 80 percent success after twelve weeks. Treating wounds with honey prior to skin-grafting operations was found to result in better graft uptake as well.
- In a 2004 British study, researchers experimented with honey on a group of forty patients with leg-vein ulcers caused by poor circulation that had not responded to compression bandages. For the next twelve weeks, honey dressings were applied to the leg-vein ulcers, while all other aspects of care remained unchanged. Honey reduced the pain and size of the ulcers, and the malodorous wounds were promptly deodorized.
- Similarly, honey treatment of bedsores in elderly Australian nursing-home patients resulted in rapid and complete healing and deodorization of wounds.

Healing Dermatitis and Skin Fungal Infections with Honey

Saudi Arabian physicians and medical researchers have a long-standing interest in honey. Noori Al-Waili, M.D., Ph.D., of the Dubai Specialized Medical Center, Saudi Arabia, is an expert on medicinal honey. In one study, he treated thirty-seven patients with skin fungal infections with a salve of equal parts honey, olive oil, and beeswax for up to four weeks. The patients were infected with pityriasis versicolor, tinea cruris, tinea corporis, or tinea faciei. These parasitic fungi live on the skin surface, or just below the surface, and cannot be scraped or washed off.

Honey, olive oil, and beeswax salve is an ancient Middle Eastern treatment mentioned in both the Bible and the Koran. For each fungal disease, the percentage of patients cured ranged from 62 to 86 percent. Redness, scaling, itching, and burning were all improved, and in some cases the fungi were fully eradicated.

Atopic Dermatitis
A condition of chronic allergic skin rashes, itching, and irritation that occurs in persons with a genetic susceptibility to allergies. Allergies to eggs, wheat, pet dander, or laundry soaps often can cause atopic dermatitis.

In a subsequent study, Dr. Al-Waili used the same preparation to treat patients with *dermatitis* and *psoriasis*. Twenty-one patients with dermatitis and eighteen patients with psoriasis were treated on one side of the body with the honey-olive oil-beeswax salve. The other side was treated with petroleum jelly mixed with a standard steroid drug.

More than half of the patients responded well to the honey-olive oil-beeswax treatment in just two weeks. Their skin softened and was less red and itchy. In addition, all the patients were able to reduce their steroid drug doses by 75 percent without experiencing flare-ups. And once again, the honey treatment cost less and had no side effects compared to standard drug therapy.

Treating Gastrointestinal Disorders with Honey

Honey was a remedy for indigestion, diarrhea, and various stomach pains throughout the ancient world. Stomach ulcers, heartburn, and dypepsia (chronic indigestion) are considered to be wounds of the body's interior tissues.

Manuka honey has been anecdotally recommended for stomach and duodenal ulcers. (The duodenum is a portion of the intestines attached to the base of the stomach.) Case reports from physicians in New Zealand report that it is effective. In cell cultures, manuka honey has been shown to inhibit the growth of *Helicobacter pylori,* the bacteria that often causes or contributes to the development of stomach ulcers and dypepsia. Manuka honey is active against other gastrointestinal bacteria also, including *Escherichia coli* and *Streptococcus faecalis.*

Animal studies with mixed floral honey from Saudi Arabia showed that it both prevented the formation of stomach ulcers and healed existing ones in rats. Ulcers were induced by alcohol (ethanol) or aspirin and related drugs. To gain protection, the rats needed to ingest honey thirty minutes prior to drinking ethanol, but they could take honey in advance or along with drugs and still be protected.

In another study, honey given to rats at 5 grams (gm) per kilogram (kg) of body weight afforded 100 percent protection from experimental colitis. Colitis was induced by putting strong acetic acid in the rats' stomachs. A sugar mixture of glucose, fructose, sucrose, and maltose was also tested but had no protective effect compared to real honey.

In a 1981 human clinical trial, the Saudi mixed floral honey was the sole medication given to forty-five patients with dyspepsia. Each patient took 30 ml honey prior to meals three times a day for a month. Only eight patients reported little or no relief.

Dr. Al-Waili, the Saudi expert on medicinal honey mentioned earlier, found that eating honey daily specifically reduces biochemicals associated with inflammation (prostaglandins) in healthy men and women. The effect of honey on prostaglandin levels was found to be cumulative, that is, prostaglandin levels were lower after fifteen days than one day whereas a sugar mixture of glucose, fructose, sucrose and maltose had the opposite effect of *increasing* prostaglandins.

Plant species known to be sources for the Saudi honeys used in the animal and human studies were acacia, juniper, mulberry, and indigo. Interestingly, honey from bees fed sugar water was far less effective than the natural floral honey.

In another trial, honey was shown to be effective for pediatric infectious gastroenteritis. This condition causes diarrhea, vomiting, and fever and is a major worldwide health problem. In this study, 169 infants and children with gastroenteritis were assigned to receive a rehydration solution containing either 5 percent honey or 5 percent glucose (the standard treatment). All the infants and children treated with the honey solution recovered as well, or better than, those who received the glucose solution. A subgroup of infants and children, who had been diagnosed with bacterial infections, recovered in an average time of fifty-eight hours if given honey compared to ninety-three hours if given glucose.

How Does Honey Work Medicinally?

Raw honey is preferred for both consumption and medicinal use. In contrast to pasteurized honey, raw honey is extracted from the comb with a minimum of processing and is not overheated or sterilized. It contains active enzymes, vitamins, and volatile chemical constituents that are destroyed or removed by high heat and processing.

There are five major reasons for the wound healing properties of honey:

1. All honey is 15 to 21 percent water with most of the remainder consisting of the sugars glu-

cose and fructose. These sugars are strongly attracted to the water and bond to it to form a syrup. This property is valuable because a layer of honey when placed over a wound will absorb body fluids, thus desiccating bacteria and fungi, and inhibiting their growth. This is the primary reason why honey clears infections in wounds so fast.

2. *Only* raw honey produces hydrogen peroxide in the presence of water or water-rich fluids. This is due to the action of the enzyme glucose oxidase, which the bees secrete into the honey.

   Glucose oxidase is only activated in the presence of water. This means that raw honey in the jar does not produce hydrogen peroxide, but when the honey comes into contact with body fluids leaking from an open wound, the enzyme is activated. Interestingly, the activity of glucose oxidase *increases* when honey is diluted, so this action of honey keeps working on a wound that is weeping.

   Hydrogen peroxide is a powerful antiseptic and anti-inflammatory. While hydrogen peroxide can be helpful for sterilizing a wound in the initial stages of healing, it irritates tissues and prevents healing when continually used on wounds.

   In contrast, the glucose oxidase in honey produces small but steady amounts of hydrogen peroxide. With nature in charge, the miniscule amount produced is just enough to sterilize wounds and stimulate tissue repair, but not enough to interfere with healing. It's the "slow drip" method of giving the body what it can use at once, but no more. And, of course, if the wound heals and dries up, glucose oxidase can't work so no unneeded peroxide is produced.

Keep in mind that all the naturally occurring enzymes in honey are destroyed by pasteurizing and heating, improper storage, and bright light, so the ability to make hydrogen peroxide is lost in many commercial honeys.

3. Floral honey contains additional healing and anti-infective compounds, which vary depending on the plants from which the honey originated. In a study of 345 unpasteurized honey samples, the majority exhibited antibacterial action against *Staphylococcus aureus,* a major cause of serious wound infections. After all the glucose oxidase was neutralized so that the effects of hydrogen peroxide were removed, only honey from manuka (*Leptospermum scoparium*) and viper's bugloss (*Echium vulgare*) plants were still active in a significant proportion of samples.

   Stronger, darker honeys and those from aromatic plants have greater antioxidant and antimicrobial activity. Mixed desert, sage, thyme, eucalyptus, manuka, and buckwheat honeys are good, readily available choices for medicinal use. In India, lotus honey is revered for healing, as is neem honey in Indonesia.

4. Honey is an anti-inflammatory. Wounds that are not healing well almost always have chronic inflammation. You have probably seen an angry red ring and a "doming up" of tissue around a wound. Inflamed wounds cause pain, burning, and itching.

   Chronic wound inflammation may be a result of lingering bacterial or fungal infections. It may also be a result of consistent pressure such as in bedsores, or poor circulation caused by diabetes or varicose veins. Chronic inflammation and slow healing of wounds and injuries can also be a problem when a person's immune system is compromised.

Honey's antioxidants counteract the irritating effects of excess ROM production, which helps wounds heal more cleanly and promoting healthy new tissue growth. Some of the essential oil components in honey also act as anti-inflammatories.

5. All raw honey contains varying amounts of propolis and bee pollen. Propolis and pollen always contain a full spectrum of vitamins, *trace elements*, and phytochemicals. Many of these are antimicrobial and are known to stimulate the growth of healthy new tissue. The healing aspects of propolis and bee pollen are discussed in upcoming chapters.

Trace Element
The scientifically correct term for single element essential minerals such as calcium, copper, iron, and zinc that we need in doses less than one gram per day.

Purchasing and Using Honey at Home

Despite these incredible medical benefits, honey is mainly purchased for its sweet taste. Honey in general, and especially raw honey, is nutritionally superior to white, brown, and "raw" cane or beet sugars, fructose, and fruit sugar extracts. The sugars in honey are easily digested, and the vitamins, minerals, and enzymes present in raw honey aid digestion and metabolism.

Phytochemicals from the various nectar source plants cause endless variation in honey. Raw unprocessed or lightly processed honey retains the flavor and aroma of the nectar source plants, but it is highly variable. Highly processed "supermarket" honey is pleasantly sweet and homogeneous, but is also bland and generic. Medicinally and nutritionally, raw honey in the best choice, therefore it's a good idea to start your children on raw honey at an early age so that their palates become educated to flavors beyond just "sweet."

One way to learn which honeys appeal to you is to visit a natural food store or farmer's market in an area known for apiculture. Keep in mind that you may want to purchase strong, dark, aromatic honeys for medicinal use, and lighter honeys for table use.

After opening, honey can be stored sealed, and out of direct heat and light, at room temperature for at least four to six months. A kitchen cabinet is a good storage location. However, if you buy honey in bulk, or the weather or climate is hot, you may want to keep a small jar on the shelf and refrigerate the remainder until needed. If you have ants in your home, honey may need to be stored in the refrigerator or inside a larger container with a screw-on lid.

If honey crystallizes in your jar, heat it for five to fifteen seconds on high in the microwave, and the crystals will readily melt. Keep the jar lid on loosely to prevent splattering. Or put the whole sealed jar in a boiling water bath on the stove. Watch carefully and remove it when it has liquefied.

Precautions for Ingesting Honey

Since approximately 80 percent of honey consists of glucose and fructose, honey is a concentrated source of simple sugars. Excessive consumption is not recommended for anyone with diabetes, abnormal glucose tolerance, hypertension (high blood pressure), or obesity.

On occasion honey can cause allergic reactions, and unfortunately such reactions are most commonly observed when raw, unprocessed honey is consumed. The allergic reactions are due the small amounts of certain phytochemicals, pollen, and/or bee dander in the honey and not to the sugars. Sometimes switching to another variety of honey or using processed honey solves the problem, but if you've been allergic to one honey, *always* use caution when trying others.

Children under twelve months of age should not be fed raw *or* pasteurized honey unless under medical supervision, as in the study of childhood gastroenteritis mentioned above. Although honey is relatively sterile, some hardy bacterial and fungal spores can occur and survive pasteurization. Pasteurized honey cannot be heated to very high temperatures, since this would destroy the honey. While the minor amount of spores in honey poses no risk for adults or even toddlers, small infants may suffer serious infections—in particular botulism.

Botulism is caused by a virulent toxin from the bacterium *Clostridium botulinum,* which naturally exists in soils. Botulism spores enter lots of foods from soil and dust contamination, but they can't germinate when heated to boiling temperatures, or in acid conditions (below pH 4.6), or with high amounts of sugar, so they don't actually germinate in honey—or in most other foods. They also don't germinate inside adult humans or children, because our stomach acid kills them.

However, young infants don't produce strong stomach acid like children and adults do, thus spores can germinate in their intestines. Approximately 95 percent of infantile botulism cases reported have occurred in infants under thirty-five weeks of age. However, far more cases of infantile botulism reported are from breast milk and corn syrup than from honey ingestion.

Honey used topically to treat minor wounds and infections does not pose a botulism risk unless it can be licked off. For infants, use large bandages that fully envelope the wounds, and don't apply honey to the baby's fingers or toes.

Treating Wounds at Home

When treating wounds at home, I often use raw, high desert honey with bee pollen added because it heals promptly and is not too runny under the bandage. Raw, comb honey with wax and propolis is also an excellent choice for first-aid because it is thick when applied and tends to stay in place on the wound. The wax and propolis work with the honey to form a protective antimicrobial seal on the wound.

To apply, simply dip a clean stick or small utensil into the honey and cover the wound with an even layer. Dress the wound with a bandage large enough that the honey will not squeeze out. Change the bandage twice a day for fresh minor wounds, and three times a day for large wounds or wounds that have become infected or have not healed well.

It is good practice to soak wounds for five to ten minutes in *hot* water with 2 tablespoons salt per gallon each time you change the dressing for the first few days after you are injured, or for three to four days after you notice a wound is infected. Make sure the water is hot enough that you must "ease" into it. Soaking wounds in hot salt water is the only standard medical practice that reliably cures external infections caused by antibiotic-resistant bacteria.

For stubborn wounds or skin ulcers I have developed the following special treatment. This treatment also works wonders on sore, weeping, inflamed burns and blisters that have had the skin torn off.

1. Mix two tablespoons room-temperature raw honey with a few teaspoons colostrum powder in a small dish to form a smooth but stiff paste. Colostrum is secreted by the mammary gland (breast or teat) in the first forty-eight hours after giving birth. It is a concentrate of immune and growth factors filtered out of the mother's blood. Colostrum gives the newborn's immune system a "jump start." Human babies get colostrum if breast-fed, and calves

always do (the bovine colostrum we use comes from cows). Manuka or eucalyptus honey are good choices for this treatment, but not strictly necessary. You can also add six drops total of manuka, tea tree, eucalyptus, and/or lavender essential oils to the mix. Lavender is especially soothing for burns.

2. Pack the paste onto the wound and bandage as described above. Your wound will not stick to the dressing, and will heal promptly with little scarring if you use this salve for four to seven days, changing the dressing and soaking the wound at least twice a day. If you do nothing else, make sure that you go to sleep each night with a clean wound and a fresh dressing. Let the miracle of honey work while you sleep.

Note: If you have a condition that suppresses immunity or reduces circulation, you must also consult a professional if wounds don't heal.

CHAPTER 2

Propolis— An Antioxidant Powerhouse

Propolis consists mainly of resins exuded from the leaf buds and bark of certain trees. The resins are collected by worker bees that specialize in harvesting resins. These workers mix the resins with a little wax, honey, and enzymes to make propolis. The honeybee colony uses propolis as putty to seal cracks and openings in the hive, and to strengthen and repair honeycombs. Propolis is also used to embalm or "mummify" the carcasses of larger animals that have invaded the hive.

Propolis helps sterilize the hive, inhibiting the spread of bacteria, viruses, and fungi that are a significant threat in such humid, close quarters. This makes good sense when you think of how illness spreads on ships or in barracks. Some bees practice preventive hygiene by lining brood cells with propolis.

Propolis has been used for humans and livestock as an antiseptic, antimicrobial, and detoxifier for over 2,000 years. European, Asian and Middle-Eastern cultures used propolis to heal festering wounds, such as bedsores, skin ulcers, and jagged battlefield slashes from bayonets. As weapons of war, bayonets were designed to produce wounds that were difficult to suture and didn't heal cleanly, and thus readily became infected.

The Origin of Propolis

Most modern research has been conducted on propolis from north temperate, mid-latitude, mixed deciduous (leafy) and evergreen forests.

These are the forest types found in northern and central Europe, northern United States, southern Ontario and Quebec, British Columbia, and Maritime Canada. The source trees are mainly from the Poplar genus. Poplars reliably exude a sticky resin called "balsam" from leaf buds. Resins from various conifers, beech, chestnut, birch, and aspen trees are also used for propolis to a lesser extent.

Propolis collected from the United States, Canada, northern and Mediterranean Europe, West Asia, southern Brazil, Uruguay, China, and New Zealand is mainly poplar-based. In far northern Russia, for example, poplars phase out and propolis comes mainly from birch and aspen trees.

Honeybees in tropical South and Central America, Hawaii, Africa, Southeast Asia, and Australia collect propolis from the native vegetation, which is nothing like that of temperate forests. Poplars are not native to these areas. Studies of tropical Brazilian propolis have identified *Eucalyptus sp.*, *Baccharis sp.*, *Araucaria sp.*, and *Hyptis divaricata* as source trees. Honeybees were introduced to Hawaii only about 100 years ago, but they quickly learned to use flowering *Plumeria* shrubs for propolis. Similarly, Venezuelan bees harvest flowering *Clusia* shrubs.

Propolis Is a Medicinal Plant

Propolis is a complex natural substance that contains hundreds of chemical compounds. Chemical analysis has focused its attention on about thirty abundant but unique constituents. This overview approach provides a chemical "fingerprint" that appears consistently in propolis analyses from a given area. This fingerprint is often an exact match with resin beads collected directly from local trees. Bees are exceedingly selective, for example, propolis collected in the Arizona Sonora desert was from only a single poplar species, *Populus fremontii.*

Propolis is approximately 50 percent resins, 30 percent waxes, 10 percent essential oils, 5 percent pollen, and 5 percent plant debris. Chemical fingerprint matching shows that bees do not make significant changes to harvested resin. Since the changes are minor, propolis is considered an herbal medicine, similar to other medicinal resins such as boswellia, guggul, and myrrh.

With detailed investigation, researchers found a subset of compounds in propolis that have a recurrent pattern of antiseptic, antibiotic, antifungal, anti-inflammatory, and detoxifying properties. Most of these compounds have been identified and studied in other medicinal plants.

Since each bee colony harvests resins from its local area, the composition of propolis varies extensively, but the medicinal properties do not. Bees have an agenda to protect their colony, and thus seek out plants that do this effectively—all over the world!

Propolis Extracts: Pros and Cons

Scientific research on propolis is limited to fractions soluble in laboratory solvents. Further, in order to be used as a dietary supplement, only water, ethanol (the alcohol we drink), or glycerol extraction is permitted. Much of the propolis material is not soluble in water, ethanol, or glycerol; therefore, whole propolis products in which the propolis is finely ground may have benefits that aren't apparent in extracts.

Both extracts and whole propolis capsules or tablets have their advantages and disadvantages. A disadvantage of extracts is that they contain only the soluble fraction, not the whole propolis material; an advantage is that the soluble portion is more likely to be absorbed.

A disadvantage of whole, encapsulated propolis is that some of the propolis cannot be absorbed, even by healthy humans and animals. Even chemical compounds that are known to be absorbable may be rendered unavailable to the body if they are bound up in a gummy, waxy, resin bead.

To use an analogy, suppose you melted sugar together with plastic and then cooled it to make a disc. If you then swallowed the disc, it would be hard for your body to extract and use the sugar because it is bound up in indigestible plastic. Shredding the disc into small pieces first could help you digest the sugar, because there is more surface area exposing sugar particles.

All discussions of propolis research need to identify the propolis source and the type of extraction. In this book, the word "propolis" refers to propolis from temperate mixed forests. Propolis from specialized locations will be identified.

Now that you are aware of the caveats, let's see what tremendous benefits propolis from all over the world has to offer!

Antibiotic Uses of Propolis

Commonly prescribed antibiotics that we have relied on for more than fifty years are rapidly becoming ineffective. Their overuse and the inevitable mutations of bacteria into resistant strains are once again turning simple infections into life-threatening illnesses. This crisis has largely been brought on by the increasing demand for antibiotics from doctors, patients, and the livestock industry, and a pharmaceutical industry that is all too willing to provide these drugs for human and animal use.

In the field of nutritional medicine, our first line of defense is a strong offense. Instead of waiting for infections to start and then utilizing a pharmaceutical approach to kill bacteria, we prefer to prevent or lessen the incidence of disease in the first place. Using propolis is something you can do right now to help combat antibiotic-resistant bacteria and to improve your immunity so that you don't succumb to illness as readily.

In cell-culture tests, ethanol, acetone, dimethyl sulfoxide (DMSO) and water extracts of propolis significantly inhibited the growth of bacteria that cause many common human diseases. For some species of bacteria, DMSO extracts of Turkish propolis performed as well or better than conventional antibiotics, however, in North America, DMSO extracts cannot be sold over the counter for internal use.

Propolis is most effective against pathogenic Gram-positive bacteria, including *Staphyloccocus sp.* (causes wound and urinary tract infections), *Clostridium sp.* (cause gastrointestinal distress), *Corynebacterium diptheriae* (causes diphtheria), and some *Streptococcus* sp. (causes strep throat, sinus infections, and scarlet fever). Propolis generally has limited activity against Gram-negative bacteria, but significantly inhibits *Klebsiella pneumonia* (causes pneumonia and bronchitis) and *Pseudomonas sp.* (causes wound infections). It is mildly active or inactive against Gram-negative *Escherichia coli, Shigella sp.* (causes dysentery) and *Salmonella sp.* (causes gastrointestinal distress).

Gram-positive and Gram-negative
A stain developed by Dr. Hans Gram for differentiating microorganisms. Microorganisms appear violet if they take up the stain (Gram-positive) and pink if they do not (Gram-negative).

Respiratory Infections

Propolis has been shown to be active against bacteria cultured directly from people with upper respiratory tract infections (the nasal passages, sinuses, and throat), including strains resistant to penicillin. It can also potentiate the action of pharmaceutical antibiotics, including streptomycin, penicillin, neomycin, chloramphenicol, and tetracycline.

A breakthrough study was published in a 2004 issue of the *Archives of Pediatric and Adolescent Medicine*. In this experiment, an Israeli research group studied the effectiveness of a syrup containing echinacea, propolis, and vitamin C in preventing respiratory tract infections in children. For twelve weeks in winter, 430 children, ages one to five years, randomly received the herbal preparation or a placebo. The following dosages were given twice daily: children ages one to three received 250 mg echinacea, 250 mg propolis, and 50 mg vitamin C; children ages four to five, 375 mg echinacea, 375 mg propolis, and 75 mg vitamin C.

There was a 55 percent reduction in the incidence of respiratory tract infections in children taking the echinacea/propolis preparation compared to the placebo (138 versus 308 infections). With the herbal preparation, the number of infections each child got was reduced by 50 percent. The duration of each illness was shorter also—the number of days each child ran a fever was reduced by 62 percent. Overall, the children who received the herbal preparation had fewer days of illness because they became ill less often, and the durations of illness episodes were shorter.

Other positive study findings support the benefits of using propolis for respiratory infections:

- In a 1997 Dutch study, mice were nasally infected with *Klebsiella pneumoniae*. Infected mice fed a propolis ethanol extract daily were three times as likely to survive the resultant pneumonia.
- In a 1995 Romanian study, preschool children had fewer incidences of upper respiratory infections and less severe symptoms when treated preventively with a commercial ethanol extract of propolis for five months.

- Case studies in Poland in the last fifty years indicate that propolis helps clear acute bronchitis and sinusitis. When propolis was combined with immune-stimulating drugs, it potentiated the effects of the medications for chronic bronchitis patients.

While studies have shown the effectiveness of propolis in preventing and reducing the severity of respiratory infections, propolis *alone* cannot be recommended for internal use as an antibiotic. If you have an *existing* respiratory infection, propolis can be taken in conjunction with antibiotic drugs, but not in place of them.

From personal experience, I recommend taking 4 to 8 grams propolis a day to help clear upper respiratory infections. Propolis is *crucial* if your infection isn't responding to prescribed antibiotics. During cold and flu season, I take 500 mg propolis a day as a preventive measure, as part of a comprehensive supplement plan. I take 1,000 mg a day when taking airline flights, or tending or visiting sick persons. Also, don't neglect to take at least 1,000 mg vitamin C one to two times daily when healthy, and three to four times daily when ill or stressed. Propolis and vitamin C are synergistic!

Keeping Teeth and Gums Healthy

Mouth rinses containing propolis are astringent and inhibit the growth of common oral bacteria. These bacteria cause halitosis, periodontal disease (gingivitis and periodontitis), tooth decay, gum disease, and poor healing after oral surgery. Propolis effectively kills oral bacteria, does not irritate teeth or gums, and is nontoxic to the tooth pulp.

Streptococcus mutans bacteria cause cavities and plaque. Plaque is an insoluble film of sugar-linked molecules that bacteria secrete in order to adhere to the tooth surface. Brazilian propolis was shown to inhibit an enzyme bacteria used to link the sugars to make plaque. It also significantly inhibited the growth of *Streptococcus mutans, Streptococcus sanguinis, and Streptococcus sobrinus*—all implicated in cavity formation.

In a 1996 Israeli study, ten dental patients were shown to have significant reductions in the levels of *Streptococcus mutans* after using a propolis oral rinse.

Water-ethanol extracts of Brazilian propolis have proven especially effective against four types of bacteria commonly associated with periodontal disease. These dangerous bacteria proliferate in the gum pockets of persons with gingivitis, and are hard to control once they get a foothold. In studies, Brazilian propolis dramatically inhibited bacterial growth in 0.05 to 0.5 percent solutions—an amount easily accommodated in standard mouthwashes.

Saliva is naturally protective against oral bacteria. Persons with "dry mouth," a condition in which there is not enough saliva in the mouth, have accelerated rates of tooth decay and periodontal disease. In a 1999 study, rats without salivary glands developed fewer cavities when their teeth were painted with Brazilian propolis twice daily.

In a 1994 Japanese study, researchers divided twenty-seven, oral, plastic-surgery patients into three groups. Group A used no mouth rinse; Group B used a 5 percent alcohol rinse and Group C, a 5 percent propolis-alcohol rinse. All groups rinsed daily and had period check-ups for forty-five days after surgery. The researchers found that patients using the propolis rinse had faster, cleaner wound healing, and a greater reduction of pain and inflammation compared to those in Groups B and C.

Propolis toothpastes and mouthwashes are

readily available. If you can't find something you like, add an entire bottle of propolis extract (ethanol-based is best) to any 24–36 ounce bottle of mouthwash.

Healing Wounds and Stimulating New Tissue Growth

In addition to preventing infection, propolis can stimulate the growth of new tissue. Researchers have found that external wounds heal faster and more cleanly if they are treated with propolis salves. Internally, case reports and animal studies indicate that propolis can help heal stomach ulcers.

In one study, Brazilian propolis cream was compared with a silver sulfadiazine salve (SS) in the treatment of minor burns. Patients in a burn clinic had propolis cream applied to one wound and SS applied to another. They returned to the clinic every three days for dressing changes. Patients did not disturb their dressings at home.

No difference in microbial growth was observed between the two treatments, however, the wounds that had been treated with propolis consistently showed less inflammation and more rapid closure. If dressings had been changed more frequently, the antimicrobial and wound healing effects of propolis would have been enhanced.

Using Propolis to Heal Skin Wounds

Everyone suffers from minor cuts, sores, and abrasions from time to time. Popular medical opinion and advertising advocate the immediate use of petroleum jelly ointments containing topical antibiotics. This approach to skin wound treatment is flawed and possibly dangerous. Constant, casual use of antibiotic ointments promotes the growth of resistant skin bacterial strains just like the overuse and misuse of oral antibiotics does in the bloodstream.

Keep in mind that a fresh, minor flesh wound is not yet infected, and so does not yet need antibiotics!

The complex blend of compounds in propolis (and other medicinal plants) is superior to a single antibiotic in petroleum jelly. It's far more difficult for pathogens to develop resistance to complex, variable substances. For example, when *Staphyloccocus aureus,* one cause of wound infections and boils, was cultured with low (nontoxic) levels of propolis extract for forty months, no resistant strains developed.

You can't get a better wound dressing than raw honey and propolis. Just open a propolis capsule and mix the powder in with a little honey, or sprinkle the propolis right on the wound.

Powdered propolis may be preferable to propolis extract for wound care because the gummy polymer that remains after extraction may gently seal off the wound. You can open a capsule or grind up a tablet in a mortar. This helps prevent infection and protects the area from further damage while new skin is forming. This sealing action really works in my experience.

Propolis salves or honey with propolis are safe for children. And don't forget your pets! Dogs and cats won't enjoy licking a propolis salve off their wounds (especially if it contains tea tree or manuka oils) like they enjoy petroleum jelly. Honey isn't a good choice for wounds that can be licked unless it has healing but distasteful herbs added.

Antifungal Actions of Propolis

Propolis inhibits the growth of wood-rotting fungi in the forest. The trees from which propolis originates manufacture resin precisely to protect themselves from such infections. Similarly, propolis can inhibit the growth of fungi that infect humans surficially. Surficial infections occur on the skin and scalp.

Propolis helps control *Microsporum sp.*, a fungus that causes ringworm, and tropical skin and scalp fungal diseases, and *Trichtophyton sp.*, a fungus that causes most skin and nail infections. Propolis is not considered very effective against subcutaneous (below the skin or deeply embedded in the skin and nails) or systemic (internal) fungi.

In cell cultures, some types of propolis inhibit the growth of *Candida albicans,* the culprit in common "yeast" infections. Propolis has been effective when used topically for vaginal and oral *Candida* infections. However, internal use of propolis is not reliably effective in alleviating chronic, systemic yeast infections.

Persons with AIDS have greatly compromised immune systems and are unable to prevent infections from fungi and bacteria that are harmless to healthy people. Propolis has been very successful in treating persistent skin and mouth infections caused by immune suppression. One such infection is oral *Candida,* also called "thrush."

The Brazilian AIDS community is largely responsible for bringing Brazilian propolis to the forefront of medicine. (In Brazil, propolis is also taken internally for AIDS because it has some ability to reduce replication of the HIV virus.)

In a 2002 study, twelve *Candida* strains were collected from a group of Brazilian HIV-positive patients with thrush. The strains were tested against a commercial Brazilian propolis ethanol extract and four standard antifungal drugs (nystatin, clotrimazole, econazole, and fluconazole). The *Candida* strains were inhibited equally well by propolis and nystatin, but showed resistance to the other drugs.

When patients with chronic sinusitis caused by *Candida* sprayed an alcohol-oil emulsion of propolis into their nostrils after daily saline irrigation, nine of twelve patients fully recovered, and three improved significantly in ten to seventeen days. Note that propylene glycol, alcohol, or DMSO extracts are useful for treating fungal infections. Water- and glycerol-propolis extracts, however, are ineffective. Please consult a doctor or health-care practitioner for treatment of fungal infections because they can be very difficult to cure.

Antiviral Uses of Propolis

In cell cultures, propolis inhibits the growth and replication of viruses, including polio, herpes, influenza, adenovirus (colds), and rotavirus (stomach flu). For centuries propolis has been a primary treatment for viral infections, but there are few human studies to support these findings.

The studies mentioned previously in which propolis helped prevent respiratory infections also support propolis's antiviral action, because many of the infections it prevented were adenoviruses. Another breakthrough study (discussed next) was published in 2000, which clearly supports topical use of propolis for genital herpes.

Herpes Simplex Infection

Ninety men and women with recurrent genital herpes infections participated in a study at Lvov State Medical University in the Ukraine. After they had an outbreak, the patients reported to the clinic to receive one of three treatments: a Canadian propolis ointment with 3 percent propolis; an acyclovir drug ointment with 5 percent acyclovir; or a plain ointment (placebo). The propolis ointment was prepared by extracting propolis with ethanol and then drying off the solvent.

Patients treated their sores with the ointment four times a day for ten days. As the outbreak progresses, the lesions—which start as small bumps—open up and ulcerate. The ulceration stage is the most painful. After a few days to a week the ulcers crust over and eventually heal.

Progression of the lesions was about three

days faster in patients receiving the propolis ointment compared to patients using either the acyclovir ointment or placebo. After ten days, twenty-four of thirty patients receiving propolis had healed lesions, compared to fourteen of thirty patients using the acyclovir, and only twelve of thirty patients using the placebo. All eighteen patients who started propolis when their lesions were already in the ulceration stage were completely healed!

To treat herpes yourself, you can follow the experimental protocol above with any commercial propolis ointment or just add propolis powder to a tea tree or mauka salve.

Anti-inflammatory Actions of Propolis

Propolis ethanol, water, and DMSO extracts have demonstrated reliable anti-inflammatory effects in animals and humans. Propolis can help relieve conditions associated with inflammation such as arthritis, boils, pustular acne, asthma, dermatitis, ulcers, and inflammatory bowel diseases.

Propolis has successfully reduced inflammation in experiments on rats with various types of arthritis. In one study, physical weakness and stiffness in arthritic rats was suppressed by 50 or 100 mg/kg per day propolis-ethanol extract. Pain relief in the animals that were given the 100 mg/kg dose was comparable to the steroid prednisolone at 2.5 mg/kg per day and aspirin at 100 mg/kg per day.

It's important to realize that these doses of steroids and aspirin are very high and have severe side effects. They could not be used safely on a long-term basis. For people with arthritis or similar inflammatory conditions, using high doses of propolis is much safer.

Unique to Propolis: Caffeic Acid Phenethyl Ester

The major anti-inflammatory phytochemical in

propolis is caffeic acid phenethyl ester (CAPE). High levels of CAPE are unique to nontropical propolis. In every cell culture and animal study from 1995 to 2002, CAPE was the strongest antioxidant and anti-inflammatory compound identified in propolis. Further, if CAPE was removed from the propolis, it no longer had significant anti-inflammatory activity.

CAPE inhibits the enzyme responsible for the conversion of *arachidonic acid* to pro-inflammatory series-2 eicosanoids. Eicosanoids are hormonelike biochemicals that control activities locally where they are produced. When their job is done they quit and are "decommissioned" promptly. Eicosanoids are vital to our health, but if the production of series-2 eicosanoids is excessive or unbalanced, inflammatory conditions such as arthritis, asthma, psoriasis, and allergies are exacerbated.

Arachidonic Acid
A 20-carbon, omega-6 polyunsaturated fatty acid that is essential for all mammals.

In a 2002 Italian study, 300 mg/kg propolis-ethanol extract was as effective as 30 mg/kg isolated CAPE for treating arthritis in rats. Further, this dose of CAPE was found to be nearly as effective as 0.2 mg/kg methylprednisone, the most common steroid drug prescribed for inflammation. The propolis extract with CAPE removed was also studied, but it gave no improvement over control.

Treating Inflammation with Propolis

If you have a chronic inflammatory condition such as arthritis, tendonitis, or asthma, it may be improved over the long run by taking one to two capsules of propolis daily. However, this low dose will not provide immediate relief from pain or symptoms. Keep in mind that 100 mg/kg per day really is a hefty dose. For a 100 kg (220 pound) person, this means taking 10,000 mg per day, or 10 grams.

Propolis doses of 3 to 5 grams (or the equivalent of 3 to 5 droppers of liquid) daily will be required to reduce pain associated with chronic inflammation. After four to six weeks, you can reduce this dose by half if you are having good results.

For treating acute inflammatory conditions such as sports injuries, stings, sprains, hay fever, or sinusitis, use 4 to 7 grams or 4 to 7 droppers of liquid a day for three to six days.

Note: Please consult your doctor or healthcare professional if acute inflammation continues unabated for ten days or more.

Detoxifying Actions of Propolis

Propolis ethanol extracts or propolis ethanol water extracts have strong antioxidant and detoxifying activity. For example, two generations of mice fed chow supplemented with propolis lived longer than controls fed standard rodent chow. The researchers suggested that the increased lifespan was due to the antioxidant effect of propolis.

Propolis is comparable or superior to other herbal antioxidants and detoxifying supplements on the market.

Findings from studies in Cuba, India, and Egypt concluded that treatment with propolis reduces liver damage in rats given carbon tetrachloride, a dry-cleaning solvent. Carbon tetrachloride is a toxic chemical that causes fatal oxidative damage and "ballooning" of liver cells. The rats exhibited a significant elevation of liver enzymes, an indication that the detoxifying capability of their livers was highly stressed. When propolis extract was coadministered with carbon tetrachloride, it greatly reduced oxidative damage, enzyme levels, and cell ballooning in the liver.

Keep in mind these animals were exposed to deadly levels of toxins all at once, overwhelming the liver's ability to detoxify. It is likely that detoxification of the low levels of toxins to which we are exposed to daily could be accomplished with lower intakes of propolis. Consider it "preventing" poisoning, not treating it after the fact. To take propolis as a daily preventative, see the dosage recommendations under "How to Purchase and Use Propolis" at the end of this chapter.

Dioxin-type chemicals from hazardous waste sites do not become highly toxic to us until they make a change one of the receptors (aryl hydrocarbon or AhR) on our cell membranes. This change renders the receptor dysfunctional so that biochemicals that should bind to the receptor no longer do. Losing active AhR strongly interferes with our metabolisms, causing cancer, birth defects, immune suppression, and liver, thymus, and kidney disease.

It's been observed that many fruits and vegetables we commonly eat, such as carrots, spinach, broccoli, cabbage, tomatoes, blueberries, grapes, sweet potatoes, and garlic can partially prevent this damage to AhR. This is *exactly how* phytochemicals "detoxify" dioxins—they make it such that these toxic pollutants can't readily do their dirty work. Brazilian propolis is about ten times as effective as spinach or broccoli and approximately 100 times as effective as grapes or sweet potatoes in suppressing damage to AhR. Propolis is one of the most powerful phytochemical detoxifiers known.

How Does Propolis Work Medicinally?

There are seven major reasons why propolis is so effective:

1. More than 180 phytochemicals in propolis are known to have biological activity in humans. Propolis contains flavonoids, organic acids and their derivatives, *phytosterols,* and terp-

enoids (essential oil compounds). Many of these compounds have long lists of biological activities, including anti-inflammatory, antimicrobial, antimutagenic, antihistamine, and antiallergenic properties, and are found in numerous medicinal plants.

Phytosterols
Fat-soluble phytochemicals composed of four-linked nonphenolic rings that can mimic human steroids such as cholesterol and sex hormones.

2. Flavonoids are the most abundant compounds in propolis. As explained in Chapter 1, flavonoids are especially potent antioxidants. Pinocembrin, pinostrobin, galangin, quercetin, kaempferol, apigenin, naringenin, fisetin, rhamnetin, luteolin, tectochrysin, and various hydroxychalcones are a few examples of the many flavonoids in propolis.

   Clinically, propolis is considered to stimulate the growth of new tissue in addition to preventing infection. Quercetin, kaempferol, apigenin, and luteolin in particular are known to have tissue-strengthening and regenerative effects, as well as antinflammatory and antiallergenic properties. In fact, these four flavonoids are reported to have ten to fifty pharmacological and biological activities each!

3. Other phytochemicals identified in propolis have antibiotic activity, including the organic acids and their derivatives cinnamic, ferulic, benzoic, caffeic, and coumaric; terpenes and their derivatives limonene, p-cymene, eugenol, 1,8 cineole; and the flavonoids pinocembrin, pinostrobin, galangin and quercetin.

4. Some of the same phytochemicals identified in propolis have antifungal activity, including the organic acids coumaric and caffeic acids derivatives; the terpene derivatives limonene,

1,8 cineole; and the flavonoids pinocembrin, quercetin, sakauranetin.

5. All the organic acids and their derivatives, terpenes and their derivatives, and flavonoids, identified in propolis contribute to its antiviral effects. Especially important are CAPE, quercetin, galangin, and kaempferol.

6. Propolis is rich in antioxidants, including CAPE, galangin, kaempferol, caffeic acid derivatives, and eugenol, and can reduce inflammation as well as pharmaceutical drugs.

7. Brazilian propolis is especially rich in terpenoids. It also contains the antioxidant and antimutagenic compounds p-coumaric acid, kaempferol, naringenin, isosakuranetin, and chrysin. Unique to Brazilian propolis are its high levels of cinnamic acid derivatives that have numerous biological activities.

How to Purchase and Use Propolis

Each bee colony harvests propolis from its local area, so there is great variation in the plant resins collected worldwide. For this reason, some bee propolis samples are more active than others. The bees are in charge of collecting the material, so humans have little control over the outcome. This limitation becomes easier to accept when you consider that the propolis-harvester bees are doing specialized work for us, gathering and concentrating a unique herbal material, which in all likelihood would be far too expensive and dangerous for humans to collect.

Most of the propolis sold in North American today is from China, where the costs of producing this labor-intensive material are reasonable. In clinical studies, Chinese propolis has so far proven as effective as European propolis.

Brazilian propolis is similar to Chinese and

European types, but it isn't a direct substitute. Brazilian propolis has fewer flavonoids and more terpenes than propolis from temperate areas. Most Brazilian propolis does not contain significant amounts of CAPE, and therefore it may not produce the same anti-inflammatory results. But Brazilian propolis is fully effective against bacteria, fungi, and viruses, and for promoting wound healing, detoxification, and tissue regeneration.

One or two capsules or tablets from any location can be used as a daily preventive, detoxifier, immune-booster, or anti-inflammatory. Each capsule or tablet will contain 250 to 550 mg propolis. The exact dosage is not important because propolis is so inherently variable that each batch a manufacturer processes is different; the capsule/tablet size is mainly designed for easy swallowing.

New to the marketplace are suspensions of very small propolis particles in honey or syrup designed to be taken by spoon. They combine whole ground propolis, propolis extract, and other ingredients in one palatable product. A raw honey based propolis suspension is an excellent treatment for wounds, burns, and skin infections. In addition, sweet propolis syrups are acceptable and safe for children.

CHAPTER 3

BEE POLLEN—NOTHING TO SNEEZE AT

Bee pollen consists of blended pollen grains collected by honeybees from a wide variety of plants. Worker bees travel from flower to flower, collecting pollen in special "baskets" on their legs. Workers normally collect more pollen than the colony needs, so beekeepers have devised special screens to scrape some of this pollen off as the bees enter the hive. The rounded pollen granules that you purchase are each a pollen basket from a bee's leg.

Pollen is a major food source for the bees, providing their protein, fat, vitamin, and trace element requirements. Plant nectar and honey provide the bees with carbohydrates for energy, but these are not complete food sources.

Pollen-collector bees are different workers than nectar-collector bees. Pollen-collectors visit plants that have the most nutritious and easy to collect pollens. These plants are not necessarily the same ones that nectar is collected from.

Unlike honey, bee pollen does not have a long tradition of use as a food per se. Widespread use of bee pollen as a food supplement began around World War II. However, humans have actually been eating bee pollen as long as they've been eating honey, because raw honey always contains pollen from the nectar source plants. In fact, the characteristic "flowery" taste of raw honey comes from small amounts of pollen in the honey. If honey is raw and unprocessed or minimally processed, the pollen is retained, whereas processed, filtered honey contains virtually no pollen grains.

Until after the Industrial Revolution in the late eighteenth century, sugar was a scare commodity but honey was not. A 1996 review in the *British Journal of Nutrition* concluded that pre-industrial Europeans ate about as much honey as they do sugar today—that's 15 to 30 kilograms (33 to 66 pounds) a year! Apiculture was big business in ancient Egypt, Greece, Rome, and throughout the Middle Ages to early modern times in Europe. Large professional apiaries sold affordable honey, beeswax, and propolis, and landowners kept a few hives.

So, we can safely conclude that people in the past ate far more pollen than we do now, due to their prodigious consumption of raw honey. Certainly beekeepers and their families ate considerable amounts and were the first to purposely eat bee pollen, right from their own hives. There's no doubt that bee pollen is safe for human consumption, but is it worth consuming?

Bee Pollen Is a Nutritious Food

Bee pollen consists of the male reproductive parts of seed plants, so it is a very concentrated source of nutrients. After the male pollen grains fertilize the female eggs, the resulting seeds contain all the genetic material and nutrients needed to grow a new plant. The nutritional composition of pollen is similar to a combination of dried legumes and nutritional yeast.

Protein, Vitamins, and Trace Elements in Pollen

The range of protein content in plant pollens is large. Bee pollen can contain 12 to 40 percent protein by dry weight. Pollen protein has a complete and balanced spectrum of amino acids (the chemical units that make up proteins), making it nutritionally complete for humans, other mammals, and birds.

Pollen contains every vitamin known, and is especially rich in pantothenic acid (vitamin B_5), nicotinic acid (vitamin B_3), and riboflavin (vitamin B_2). Cyanocobalamin (vitamin B_{12}) and vitamin D levels are fairly low, so pollen should not be considered an adequate source of these vitamins for humans, dogs, or cats. It is also not a suitable B_{12} supplement for vegan diets.

More than twenty-five trace elements account for 2 to 4 percent pollen by dry weight. Every trace element known to be essential for mammals is included. However, in order to use pollen as a calcium and magnesium supplement you would need to eat about one kilogram (2.2 lbs.) of pollen a day!

Fats in Bee Pollen

Bee pollen granules are 5 to 10 percent fat by dry weight. This translates to 2 to 3 grams of fat per ounce (twenty-eight grams or two rounded tablespoons). Fat is crucial to the health of honeybees.

Honeybees may actively seek pollen rich in fats. Mustard and dandelion pollens are some of the richest known, with 11.0 and 19.0 percent fat, respectively. In contrast, Australian *Eucalyptus* species have 0.43 to 4.6 percent fat, with the majority of species having less than 2 percent.

The fat content of pollen contains more free fatty acids and phospholipids than *triglycerides*. In contrast, vegetable oils pressed from seeds and nuts consist of seed storage fat that is more than 90 percent triglycerides.

The triglycerides that do exist in pollen are mainly polyunsaturated and monounsaturated, making pollen a healthy choice with

Triglycerides
Compounds composed of three, long chains of carbon atoms called "fatty acids" that are attached to a glycerol molecule.

respect to dietary fats. Corn, flax, willow, clover, and crucifers such as cabbage and broccoli have pollens that are especially rich in the omega-3 essential polyunsaturated, alpha-linolenic acid.

Phytochemical Nutrients in Pollen

Carotenoids
A class of fat-soluble phytochemicals that are composed of linked isoprene units. Examples are beta-carotene in carrots, lycopene in tomatoes, and lutein in marigolds.

In terms of its phytochemical content, bee pollen is a powerhouse—in fact, I'd call it the ultimate nutraceutical. Since pollen is the male reproductive part of plants, it contains a concentration of phytochemicals to ensure it makes viable seed. No matter where it's collected, pollen is uniformly rich in *carotenoids,* flavonoids, and phytosterols.

Bee pollen's exact phytochemical profile is variable depending on the source plants, location, climate, and season. However, the following phytochemicals are consistently reported:

- carotenoids: beta-carotene, lycopene, lutein, and zeaxanthin
- flavonoids: quercetin, isorhamnetin, kaempferol, rutin, luteolin, tricetin, myricetin, and herbacetin
- phytosterols: beta-sitosterol; various stigmasterols, lanosterols, and brassinosterols

Fresh, unheated pollen also contains numerous active enzymes, coenzymes, and hormones (including growth hormones) that are at least partially active in humans. Unlike honey, bee pollen's antioxidant activity cannot be mainly accounted for by phenolics. The antioxidant enzymes superoxide dismutase, catalase, peroxidase and glutathione peroxidase found in pollen are doing the job instead.

Although there are many benefits from using

vitamin and trace element supplements, essential nutrients provided in a food context are superior to synthetic supplements. Occasionally, people who don't perceive benefits to their health from taking standard nutritional supplements benefit demonstrably from bee pollen. These people may be unable to absorb and utilize vitamins well unless they are obtained from a food-based source. Clearly such individuals need to choose an overall nutritious diet and should consider including bee pollen.

Adding Bee Pollen to Your Diet

Bee pollen is a superior way to add servings of produce to your diet with very little effort. One teaspoon of bee pollen is equivalent to a hearty serving of vegetables. If you don't get enough chances to eat fruits and vegetables, a tablespoon of bee pollen each day is a quick and easy way to dramatically improve your diet. It's a good choice for the ill or elderly who perhaps can't cook, chew, or digest large amounts of produce.

When first trying bee pollen use fresh, soft granules, and eat only a few at a time to make sure you are not allergic to it. Allergies to bee pollen are no more common than allergies to other foods, but they do occur. If you are allergic to bee stings, be especially cautious. If you have no adverse reaction, increase your pollen intake to one tablespoon at once. One to three tablespoons a day is a good range for long-term consumption.

Physically chewing pollen granules or tablets is the best way to eat pollen and is particularly recommended if you are dieting, since you get the full sensation of eating a nutritious food. However, if you just can't get used to the taste, mix the pollen with another food, or swallow it whole with a "chaser."

If you aren't dieting, try mixing bee pollen

granules with peanut butter or other type of nut butter, and dry milk or hot cocoa mix (you can use sugar-free). Form into balls or discs and refrigerate to harden. Also, try adding bee pollen to trail mix or granola.

Pollen can also be added to blender drinks and smoothies, but I really don't recommend this unless you *really love* the taste of pollen. A little bit of bee pollen goes a long way when blended, similar to citrus peel. Also like citrus peel, pollen become bitter when pulverized.

Sweetened, chewable pollen wafers are readily available in flavors such as orange, honey, and vanilla. These are recommended for children, or adults with a sweet tooth so strong they can't enjoy pollen "as is." Unsweetened, pressed pollen tablets are intended to be swallowed whole, not chewed. Bee pollen granules are also available encapsulated, but this is an expensive option compared to granules sold in bulk.

A few manufacturers make snack/sports nutrition bars that contain bee pollen. The disadvantage of these bars is that they normally contain less than 1 gram of pollen, whereas one tablespoon of pollen weighs at least 8 grams. The advantage is that these bars are a healthy choice for a snack and get pollen into the diets of those who would never eat it otherwise!

Animals Thrive on Bee Pollen

Most bee pollen consumed in North America is eaten by animals. Pollen added to the diets of piglets, calves, foals, and chicks has been shown to enhance growth and overall health. Pollen fed to adult horses, hens, and pet birds increases health, fertility, and egg production. In laboratory tests, mice and rats thrived on a diet of only fresh bee pollen and water for up to a year. Dogs with poor skin and coat conditions improved when pollen was added to their diets.

Racehorses are fed large amounts of pollen, particularly on days prior to big events. Pollen is a high-energy food compared to grazing and allows the horses to conserve energy for racing. Horses that were "off their feed," listless, easily fatigued, and had poor coats recovered fully and rapidly when bee pollen was added to their diets.

Bee Pollen Is a Superior Animal Food

In a 1999 study, six female and six male rats of the same strain were fed only Arizona high desert bee pollen and water for twelve weeks, during which time they grew to adulthood. Six other male and six other female control rats were fed standard laboratory rodent chow. The rats could eat all they wanted, and the chow was crushed into small pieces comparable to the size of the pollen granules.

Both the male and female rats fed bee pollen were completely healthy, and they grew and acted normally. Rats of both sexes eating pollen had heavier brains than animals in the control group.

The most striking difference between the two groups was that rats fed bee pollen had much less body fat than rats fed chow. The chow-eating rats were verging on obesity at the end of twelve weeks, weighing three to four times more than rats fed bee pollen. The difference was more pronounced in males than females, which is expected since female mammals normally have smaller bodies with more body fat than males.

But did the rats weigh less because they disliked eating bee pollen? Previous studies have shown that when rodents are given chow and bee pollen side by side, they prefer the pollen. Apparently, rodents are smart enough to choose fresh, natural whole food over processed food. Perhaps there's a lesson here for us!

Bee Pollen in Your Pet's Diet

Bee pollen is sold in granules, tablets, and food supplements for dogs, cats, rabbits, ferrets, and other small mammals. Cats are obligate carnivores, which means they cannot live or reproduce without fresh animal flesh. Plant foods, including pollen, are not natural components of the feline diet, and cats have a limited ability to metabolize and detoxify phytochemicals. For this reason, cats should never be fed more pollen than the manufacturer recommends.

Dogs are more omnivorous and can usually handle a daily dose of pollen. Too much pollen can cause loose stools in dogs, so it's wise to start off with the manufacturer's recommended dose, and work up from there. Follow the same procedure for ferrets. Pet rodents can be fed pollen however you wish—use large quantities if your budget permits it.

Adding pollen to a bird's diet is known to promote growth and enhance breeding success in captivity. Bee pollen is thought to provide dietary components that birds naturally consume in the wild, but which are lacking in commercial bird foods, or even in fresh fruits and vegetables fed to the birds. In studies at Arizona State University, baby chicks were observed to preferentially peck out pollen granules when they were mixed with commercial birdseed.

Bee Pollen for Allergies and Hay Fever

Some pollens are lightweight and dry, and are designed to be dispersed by wind. Other pollens are heavier and sticky, and are designed to attach to visiting insects. Sticky pollen grains are like microscopic versions of "hitchhiker" burrs that hikers inadvertently pick up on their socks. Visiting insects and birds transfer pollen from one flower to another, thereby performing the crucial task of plant pollination. Since bee pollen is collected by bees before it is collected by humans, it consists mainly of sticky pollen.

Wind-borne pollens are responsible for most pollen allergies, not sticky pollens. Regular consumption of bee pollen can provide relief from allergies.

People often try bee pollen for the first time in an effort to help control pollen allergies, or "hay fever." The prevailing wisdom is that consuming small amounts of bee pollen over time works like a series of allergy shots by gradually desensitizing the body to pollen exposure. It's even been recommended that hay fever sufferers consume only bee pollen from their local neighborhood, presumably so they're eating the same pollen that's in the air around them.

While bee pollen can help allergies, there is no scientific evidence that it works like allergy shots, or that locally derived pollen is required or even preferred. In fact, there's little clinical evidence that allergy shots themselves are effective, especially considering the enormous time and expense that must be invested in their treatment. Let's apply some scientific logic to the use of bee pollen for allergies:

- Bee pollen is a blend of sticky pollen grains, which contain little of the windborne pollens that are widely allergenic such as ragweed, birch, olive, and grasses. Therefore, it doesn't make sense to use bee pollen to desensitize yourself to a specific airborne allergen such as ragweed pollen.

- Beekeepers primarily select locations for their hives based on the proximity to nectar source plants that produce tasty, clear honey. Secondarily, beekeepers select locations that have nutritious pollen source plants, which the bees prefer, so that the colony remains strong.

  In general, plants that are known to produce

allergenic pollen do not fit the criteria used to site beehives. The reason for this is that not all pollens are adequately nutritious for bees. For example, some of the most nutritious pollen comes from fruit trees, dandelion, willow, and clover—plants pollinated by bees. Flowering plants and bees exist symbiotically, so presumably these plants found it advantageous to produce pollen that keeps bees coming back. In contrast, corn, wheat, alder, hazel, and pine are wind-pollinated and produce pollen of inferior nutritional quality.

- Quality pollen manufacturers always blend pollen from different locations, seasons and/or source apiaries, so there's actually no consistent single local source.
- As previously stated, pollen-collector bees are different workers than nectar-collector bees. Pollen-collectors visit plants that have the most nutritious and easy-to-collect pollens. These plants are not necessarily the same ones that nectar is collected from. Although your local apiary may sell unifloral honey, this does not mean that the pollen is unifloral!
- Using very high intakes of pollen or of allergy preparations containing pollen during hay fever season helps allergies more than using very small amounts, that is, desensitizing levels throughout the year. An allergy shot contains miniscule amounts of pollen antigen compared to the amount in just a single capsule of bee pollen.
- As discussed in Chapter 2, propolis acts as an antihistamine and anti-inflammatory. Using propolis alone, or even better, along with bee pollen helps allergies.
- Bee pollen helps dust, pet dander, mold, and mildew allergies, too.

While some degree of generalized pollen desensitization activity cannot be ruled out, it's more important to focus on the large number of antiallergenic, anti-inflammatory, and immune system normalizing phytochemicals in pollen as the potential source of its allergy benefits. In this way, bee pollen functions just like other medicinal plants that are known to help allergies, asthma, and upper respiratory infections.

Using Bee Pollen to Help Your Allergies

Some of these antiallergenic, anti-inflammatory, and immune system normalizing phytochemicals were discussed in the previous chapter on propolis. The flavonoid quercetin, for example, is an antihistamine, antiallergenic, and antiasthmatic agent that is proving to be valuable for the treatment of asthma, chronic obstructive pulmonary disease, bronchitis, sinusitis, colds, flu, and allergies.

Both bee pollen and propolis contain flavonoids, carotenoids, and phytosterols with the above activities. Some of the same phytochemicals are in both products, and some are exclusive to one. Although the exact phytochemical makeup of all beehive products is dependent on the source plants, location, climate, and season, they are still effective for allergies despite variations.

Remember that bees use pollen and propolis to stay healthy themselves. They purposefully make their selections from a variety of plants, which in turn provide a variety of phytochemicals, many of which have similar activities. They intend to be redundant so that no matter the pollen blend, there are components present that will do the job. And this is true for you as well!

To treat allergies with bee pollen, select a product that contains pollen that agrees with you, because you will be using a lot of it! Start today by following the advice in the section "Adding Bee Pollen to Your Diet" mentioned earlier in the chapter. Please take at least 1,000 mg vitamin C each day also. Vitamin C is your best and safest natural antihistamine.

During allergy or "hay fever" season, triple or quadruple your daily pollen intake. Take 1,000 mg vitamin C and propolis three to five times a day along with the pollen to further help your allergies. The idea is to get enough antihistamine and antiallergenic phytochemicals into your system to make a real improvement in acute symptoms.

Some manufacturers sell special bee-pollen allergy preparations. These are fine also, but use them as directed—or even double the dosage. Again, these allergy preparations are designed to help acute symptoms. They cannot help you if you are stingy or reluctant to take more than one or two capsules a day, because this won't provide enough of the active phytochemicals and vitamins.

Precautions

Sometimes people are highly allergic to bee pollen, honey, propolis, or royal jelly and need to avoid beehive products. These people have allergic reactions that only get worse with time, and a desensitizing process can't be expected to be successful—in fact, it may be life threatening.

Persons allergic to bee pollen may have multiple pollen allergies. Honey and propolis are known to contain numerous pollen grains, and bees use pollen to make royal jelly. Mold spores in bee products are another cause of allergic reactions.

However, most people allergic to beehive products are actually allergic to the honeybee proteins. You can be allergic to "bee dander" just like you can be allergic to cat, dog, or cockroach dander. You don't have to be allergic to bee stings to be allergic to bee dander.

Other Medicinal Properties of Bee Pollen

The detoxifying and healing properties of bee pollen have been appreciated for years. Pollen has reportedly helped to combat anemia, fatigue, infertility, impotence, varicose veins, recovery from illness and surgery, prostatitis (inflammation of the prostate), high cholesterol and triglycerides, and even cancer. Adding bee pollen to the diet has been shown to stimulate the immune system. It also lowers ROM in the bloodstream and tissues.

- A 1971 study found that forty patients with bleeding gastric ulcers given 250 mg bee pollen twice a day improved remarkably.
- Chinese studies on humans and animals have demonstrated that consuming bee pollen or various single plant pollens several days prior to moving to high altitude reduces the incidence of altitude sickness and improves adaptability to lower oxygen levels.
- Standardized pollen extract was judged an effective treatment for prostate enlargement and prostatitis in two controlled clinical trials. There were no significant side effects.
- In a prolonged study, rats were exposed to organic solvent vapors thirty hours a week for three months, simulating industrial exposure. This caused a significant elevation of liver enzymes in the rats, indicating that the detoxifying capabilities of their livers were being stressed. In contrast, rats given pollen extracts had significantly lower enzyme levels than untreated rats. Exposure to the solvent also increased serum cholesterol 104 percent and triglycerides 37 percent compared to only slight increases in the control rats. Such dramatic

increases in blood lipids (fats) are another indication of liver stress.

How Does Pollen Work Medicinally?

There are five reasons for pollen's medicinal benefits:

1. Bee pollen is rich in carotenoids, flavonoids, phytosterols, and antioxidant enzymes. Many of these phytochemicals promote detoxification and act as antiviral, antibacterial, antiallergenic, anti-inflammatory, and antimutagenic agents.
2. Lycopene, beta-sitosterol and other phytosterols, and several flavonoids in pollen can reduce prostate inflammation and are associated with a lower risk of prostate cancer. Phytosterols can mimic mammalian sex hormones and are actually taken up by the prostate gland.
3. Epidemiological studies have shown that the higher your flavonoid intake, the lower your risk for cardiovascular disease. Flavonoids found in pollen are known to lower cholesterol, stabilize and strengthen capillaries, reduce inflammation, and quench ROM.
4. Rutin is a flavonoid especially concentrated in pollen that is known to improve the condition and function of capillaries. This helps to control and prevent varicose veins, venous insufficiency, hemorrhoids, hypertension, and diabetic retinopathy.
5. Bee pollen provides humans and animals with a food-based source of vitamins and trace elements. Individuals who are ill or injured often do not absorb food and nutrients as well as they should. Healing also requires higher than normal levels of nutrients. Bee pollen provides numerous essential nutrients in a concentrat-

ed, digestible form that may be superior to synthetic supplements.

How to Purchase and Store Bee Pollen

High-quality, fresh pollen should consist of soft, pliable granules that have not been pasteurized or heat-treated. Freezing pollen as it is collected and storing it frozen until packaging produces the highest-quality material. The granules should smell and taste flowery, and both sweet and tart, similar to fruit that is not quite ripe.

Quality bee-pollen manufacturers always blend pollen from different locations, seasons, and/or source apiaries. Since some plant pollens are not as nutritious or tasty as others, blending is beneficial. For example, in the rodent-feeding studies mentioned above, it was found that only four of the seven commercially available bee pollens were able to keep the mice alive for a year. Bee pollen from the southwestern U.S. desert proved to be the best choice. Mesquite trees are a major source for this pollen, but good practices in collecting, blending, and processing all contributed to the fact that this pollen was a better food.

If your first trial of bee pollen causes *mild* throat, chest, or stomach irritation, don't give up! Instead, please send it back to the manufacturer with a letter indicating that you wish to try a different lot number. You may be sensitive to only one component of the pollen blend, or even to mold spores in the pollen.

Is Bee Pollen an Organic Food?

Numerous research studies have shown that all beehive products can become contaminated with pesticides, herbicides, heavy metals, and environmental pollutants. Luckily, bees are fairly sensitive to pesticides and pollutants. The queen bee's health declines when the hive is exposed to more toxins than it can handle, so this limits the success of apiculture in heavily contaminated areas. Also, certain pesticides kill bees at levels normally used, so they aren't used much on crops that depend on bee pollination.

Quality manufacturers utilize bee pollen collected in rural or wilderness areas, away from major sources of agricultural and industrial pollution. The very best pollen comes from wild plant sources. Second best, but still excellent, is pollen from organic farming areas.

In order to utilize the "USDA Organic" label, pollen must be at least 95 percent certified organic in origin. This means that the pollen and honey from the hives in question has been analyzed and found to contain acceptably low levels of herbicides, pesticides, and heavy metals. It also means that an area well beyond the bees' source area has been certified organic.

Pollen and honey from hives that are used to pollinate mainstream commercial crops such as oranges and almonds cannot be labeled USDA Organic. In fact, it is deceptive to use the word "organic" anywhere on the label. However, many apiaries are very small businesses that may not have the time or money to become certified organic. *This does not mean that their pollen or honey is contaminated.* If you are in doubt, look for bee products that come from wild plant sources.

Pollen Processing: Pros and Cons

Some processing of pollen is necessary because the pollen grains have two tough outer coats surrounding the nutritive contents. The bees' digestive systems are designed to cope with these coats, but those of humans, cats, dogs, pigs, and small mammals are not. Birds and large grazing animals such as horses, goats, and cattle can handle the pollen coats because their systems are designed to process great quantities of vegetation and seeds.

Consequently, better manufacturers gently crack pollen before it is packaged. The digestibility of the protein and fat improves significantly when the pollen is cracked because 1) a portion of these nutrients is contained within the pollen coats; and 2) cracking the coats allows the contents of the interior to be more easily accessed during digestion.

Granules are also encapsulated, pressed into tablets or chewable wafers, or finely ground for use in foods and beverages. This may or may not damage the nutritional qualities, depending on the manufacturer. In general, American and Canadian manufacturers specializing in full-line bee products provide the freshest, highest-quality pollen.

Fresh, moist bee pollen will readily grow mold or bacteria if it is not collected off the screens regularly, and dried or frozen within about thirty-six hours of collection. For this reason, pollen collection has traditionally been more successful in warm, arid areas such as the southwestern United States and western Spain. Dried pollen does not readily support the growth of microorganisms. Bee pollen that is frozen right after it is collected is superior in taste and nutrition, and does not spoil if vacuum-packed for sale.

Pollens imported from overseas are subject to oven drying, sterilization, and longer storage durations. Excessive heating or dehydration of granules makes them hard and flinty, and can bring out a bitter taste. Oven-dried and sterilized pollens don't contain active enzymes. They can also suffer losses of vitamins, polyunsaturated fatty acids, and phytochemicals.

Storing Pollen at Home

Just like fresh produce, pollen must be handled and stored appropriately. Pollen is perishable (think of it like fresh apples) and subject to mishandling. Bee pollen sold in plastic bags should be stored in the refrigerator—before and after opening. Pollen sold in jars or in cans should always be refrigerated after opening. Any bee-pollen product can be successfully stored in the freezer. If you purchase pollen in bulk, put a small refillable container in the refrigerator for daily use, and keep the bulk of it frozen.

Pollen needs to be stored in a dark, dry environment. Never add liquids or moist foods to stored pollen, or dip damp fingers or utensils into it. Pollen that is allowed to get wet or contaminated can grow mold and/or develop off-flavors.

Bee pollen that is sold in pressed tablets or in capsules has been packaged by the manufacturer to be stored on the shelf provided that:

- the container is tightly closed after each use;
- the product is not exposed to light during storage;
- the product is used promptly;
- the storage temperature is not above 80°F.

If you can't comply with these requirements, please use your refrigerator!

CHAPTER 4

Royal Jelly—Nutrients Fit for Royalty

Royal jelly is the primary food for developing larvae in the beehive. Unlike other hive products, royal jelly is not a plant product collected and modified by bees, but a substance actually manufactured by them. Nurse worker bees ingest pollen and nectar, and then secrete royal jelly—a sort of honeybee milk—from special glands in their heads. All larvae are fed royal jelly for three days. After this the overwhelming majority of larvae are cut off from the milk because they are destined to be worker bees.

Only a few queen larvae are continually fed royal jelly. It is this rich diet of royal jelly alone that transforms the queen into a sexually mature powerhouse, living five to seven years, and laying more than her weight in eggs daily. In contrast, the worker bees are sterile and live only seven to eight weeks. The queen bee is 40 percent larger and 60 percent heavier than the workers, and is fed royal jelly throughout her life.

Taking a clue from the queen, Traditional Chinese Medicine calls royal jelly "food of the emperors." Mysterious and exotic, royal jelly was prescribed to prolong life, prevent disease, and return the vitality of youth to the aged. It remains especially prized by modern Asian cultures.

The Composition of Royal Jelly

Fresh royal jelly is roughly 66 percent water, 13 percent protein, 15 percent carbohydrate, 5 percent fat, and 1 percent trace elements. The water content normally varies from 60 to 70 percent, making royal jelly a thick, opaque, cream-colored liquid.

Phospholipids
A type of lipid that consists of two fatty-acid chains linked to a phosphate group. All our cell membranes are made of phospholipids.

Royal jelly contains all of our essential and nonessential amino acids. The carbohydrates are mostly fructose and glucose. The fat fraction contains a mix of polyunsaturated, monounsaturated, and saturated fatty acids, as well as *phospholipids.*

Royal jelly contains all the B vitamins and is particularly rich in pantothenic acid. It contains traces of vitamins A, C, D, E, and K. There are also traces of numerous phytochemicals (mainly flavonoids and phytosterols) from the pollen and nectar that the bees use to manufacture royal jelly.

While royal jelly is a balanced, nutritious food, it's not normally consumed in quantities greater than 1 or 2 grams a day. Sometimes royal jelly is recommended as a complete amino-acid supplement for vegans, or as a source of essential fatty acids. This is misleading, because the quantities of royal jelly ingested are so minute that the protein, carbohydrate, and essential fatty acid contents are inconsequential. In the majority of cases, it is more important to look at the minor components of royal jelly in order to understand its health benefits.

Minor Components of Royal Jelly

Trace constituents in royal jelly work synergistically with the nutritious base to turn an ordinary larva into a queen and greatly prolong her life.

Fresh, liquid royal jelly also contains 2.0 to 6.4 percent by weight of the short-chain fatty acid trans-10-hydroxy-2-decenoic acid (HDA). If HDA levels in a royal jelly sample are low or undetectable, then it's likely the sample has been adulterated or severely damaged during processing. Reputable manufacturers list the HDA content on the label because it's an indicator of a quality product.

Other important royal jelly constituents include:

- Collagen: The major protein of connective tissue found in skin, hair, nails, bone, cartilage, tendons, ligaments, and in the walls of our veins and arteries.
- Enzymes: Including the antioxidant enzymes superoxide dismutase, catalase, peroxidase and gluthathione peroxidase.
- Nucleic acids: DNA (deoxyribonucleic acid) and RNA (ribonucleic acid), our basic genetic building blocks.
- Gamma globulins: Natural immunizing complexes very similar to those found in human plasma. Our gamma globulins contain antibodies to the pathogens that we have been exposed to since conception.
- Methyl *p*-hydroxybenzoate (methyl paraben): A powerful antioxidant naturally present in unadulterated royal jelly that is commonly added to products as a synthetic preservative!

Royal Jelly Prevents Infection and Fatigue

Many health claims have been made for royal jelly from curing acne to reversing infertility, but almost all of these are based on anecdotal information rather than conclusive evidence from controlled studies. In case reports, royal jelly has been used successfully to treat stomach ulcers, varicose veins, impaired circulation, dyspepsia, impotence, loss of normal sexual interest, fatigue, anorexia, and viral and bacterial infections. These reports are mainly from China, Russia, and former Eastern Bloc countries.

Very little medical research is done on royal

jelly outside of Asia. This doesn't necessarily imply that fresh, high-quality royal jelly is ineffective, but rather that there hasn't been much incentive for investigation. In China, royal jelly is financially competitive with pharmaceutical medicines, so more clinical research is devoted to its use. Currently, royal jelly's reputation for returning vitality to the aged can be substantiated by controlled research showing that it helps prevent disease and alleviate fatigue.

Improves Immunity

One function of the milk that humans and other mammals produce is to help initiate normal immune responses in the newborn. Royal jelly is also considered to have this function, however, keep in mind that it's designed for developing bee larvae. The overwhelming majority of honeybees live less than two months, so the immune protection bee larvae need is minimal compared to that needed by a human infant.

Larval protection of the bee colony, however, is a different matter. Pathogens that prevent normal larval development will destroy the colony. Feeding royal jelly whether for three days to larvae destined to be worker bees or for a lifetime to the queen bee plays a role in the colony's "collective immunity." Unique proteins isolated from royal jelly are considered to be part of the honeybee's defense system against bacterial and viral infection. Here are a few highlights:

- Royalisin: One of the first proteins to be isolated, royalisin has been shown to be highly effective against eighteen types of Gram-positive, but not Gram-negative, bacteria. It was effective at very low concentrations, comparable to pharmaceutical antibiotics.
- Jellein I, II, III, and IV: In 2004 Brazilian researchers isolated these four proteins of an entirely

new class. All but Jellein IV were strongly antimicrobial, active against yeast, and both Gram-positive and Gram-negative bacteria.

- Apisin: This royal jelly glycoprotein stimulated the growth of human immune cells in culture without adding the standard cell-growth medium. Glycoproteins are proteins linked to sugars. The mucus in our nose, throat, and lungs, and most of our connective tissue is made of glycoproteins.

- Other immune-glycoproteins: Additional glycoproteins continue to be isolated from royal jelly. They are thought to be effective because bacterial cell walls are also made of glycoproteins. When we ingest harmless royal jelly glycoproteins, the body mistakes them for evidence of invading bacteria and mounts an immune response.

Royal jelly collected from three-day-old larvae has the highest quality and antimicrobial activity. In a 1995 Egyptian study, just 1 part three-day-old royal jelly in 20 parts water was shown to cause 100 percent mortality to cultures of *Staphylococcus aureus* and 71 and 83 percent mortality to cultures of *Bacillus subtilis* and *Escherichia coli,* respectively, after three hours of exposure. Mixing honey with the royal jelly potentiated this effect. *Staphylococcus aureus* could not be detected in the culture after two hours of exposure to the mixture of honey plus royal jelly.

During a flu epidemic in Sarajevo, Yugoslavia, it was reported that 9 percent of patients given royal jelly daily, developed influenza compared to 40 percent of untreated patients. Unfortunately, the dose given was not specified. The prevention of influenza may be due, at least partially, to the immune-stimulating effect of royal jelly.

Alleviates Fatigue and Stress

In a 2001 Japanese study, the endurance of mice increased when they were fed royal jelly. The royal jelly utilized was frozen immediately after collection and remained frozen until use. All the mice in the study practiced swimming in an adjustable-current pool for a few weeks.

After becoming accustomed to the regular swimming exercise, the mice were then forced to swim until exhaustion, and their times were recorded. After the swimming test, they were separated into three groups of equal endurance. Prior to their next swim, one group was given the fresh-frozen royal jelly; a second group was given royal jelly that had been stored at 40°C (124°F) for seven days; and the third group received a control solution consisting of milk protein (casein), cornstarch, and soybean oil.

The length of time mice in Group 1 could swim until exhausted was significantly longer compared to the times of Groups 2 and 3. Mice in Group 1 also showed a decreased depletion of muscle glycogen and lower blood lactic acid levels after swimming compared to Groups 2 and 3. This means that mice fed fresh-frozen royal jelly not only had more endurance, but they also were less stressed by the workout and quicker to recover after reaching exhaustion.

No significant difference in performance was observed between Group 2, which received the 40°C royal jelly, and the control group. The researchers found that a specific protein, which is utilized as a freshness marker, was degraded by heated storage.

Apparently, only fresh, unheated royal jelly has antifatigue capacity.

Royal Jelly Lowers Cholesterol and Triglycerides

A 1995 review of case-controlled human and animal studies concluded that in humans, 50 to 100 mg royal jelly (dry weight) daily decreased cholesterol by 14 percent and triglycerides by 10 percent. Most participants received injections of royal jelly, but oral doses were only slightly less effective. Royal jelly supplementation also produced these effects in animals, and slowed the development of atherosclerosis (hardening of the arteries) in rabbits fed high-fat diets.

Also in 1995, Chinese researchers reported that freeze-dried royal jelly lowered LDL or "bad" cholesterol but increased HDL or "good" cholesterol in rats with high cholesterol and triglycerides. For this experiment, animals were given 700 mg/kg per day for six weeks. This dosage also lowered the risk of developing artery-blocking clots in the bloodstream, which lead to heart attack, stroke, and phlebitis.

By 2002, the same researchers had shown that HDA was the major active compound in royal jelly responsible for producing these results. HDA isolated from royal jelly and a synthetic standard HDA both lowered cholesterol, triglycerides, and lipoproteins but raised HDL levels in rats.

It's important to bear in mind that these results were achieved in animals using 700 mg/kg royal jelly per day. The equivalent dose for a person weighing 100 kg would be 70,000 mg (70 grams) freeze-dried royal jelly per day or 210 grams of fresh royal jelly. Either amount is clearly excessive! On the other hand, supplementing with 100 mg per day is inadequate and a waste of your time and money. Exaggerated health claims for small doses of royal jelly have not been scientifically validated with controlled trials. A realistic dosage for achieving significant health improvements in adults with cardiovascular disease is 3 to 7 grams per day.

Royal Jelly Lowers Blood Pressure

In animal studies, royal jelly has effectively and safely lowered blood pressure in rats. Royal jelly itself does not have this effect, but it becomes activated by our protein digestion process. Proteins are composed of hundreds of amino acids linked together. An important step in digestion breaks protein chains down in smaller, more manageable units called peptides. Peptides have about two to ten amino acids and can be highly active.

In rats bred to develop abnormally elevated blood pressure (hypertension), a single 1.0 gm/kg dose of predigested royal jelly resulted in significant reductions of systolic (upper number on the blood pressure ratio) blood pressure. Similar effects were seen with hypertensive Chinese patients given a dosage about ten times lower, however, the studies were not controlled.

In a 2004 Japanese study with animals, predigested royal jelly doses of 0.5, 1.0, and 10 mg/kg were given to rats with genetically induced hypertension. All doses reduced systolic blood pressure for eight hours after ingestion, with the higher doses having the greater effects. After twenty-eight days, royal jelly continued to keep blood pressure under control without side effects.

Royal Jelly for the Skin

For centuries, royal jelly has been applied to soften skin, remove wrinkles, and heal eczema and dermatitis. Scientific research indicates that in concentrate form royal jelly can improve the appearance of skin and effectively treat various skin conditions. However, cosmetic and skin-care products with *traces* of royal jelly cannot be expected to provide much benefit.

As previously mentioned, collagen is the major protein in our skin. Royal jelly contains water-soluble collagen, which means that it can be directly absorbed and utilized by skin cells. Soluble collagen, an ingredient found in many cosmetic preparations, helps rejuvenate aging and damaged skin, and smooth wrinkles.

The antioxidant vitamins A, C, and E, and various carotenoids in royal jelly can also be absorbed by the skin. They work synergistically with collagen, acting to prevent skin proteins from sun and chemical damage. Individuals who have higher levels of these antioxidants in their skin—especially carotenoids—have smoother, moister skin with fewer wrinkles. They may also have a reduced risk for skin cancer.

HDA Soothes and Moisturizes Skin

Royal jelly not only contains collagen, but it may also increase the skin's natural production of collagen. When Japanese researchers isolated the component of royal jelly that was responsible for the increased production, it was none other than HDA. The more HDA the cells were exposed to, the greater the collagen production.

As noted earlier, fresh royal jelly is composed of 2.0 to 6.4 percent HDA. HDA is a 10-carbon, monounsaturated fatty acid with a single hydroxyl (OH) group on the last carbon of the chain. It's not commonly appreciated that polyunsaturated fatty acids in the skin are mainly metabolized to hydroxy fatty acids.

Let me explain the significance of this fact. Skin cells metabolize the essential polyunsaturated fatty acid gamma-linolenic acid (GLA) into its hydroxy derivative. Hydroxy-GLA protects the skin from dehydration and is strongly anti-inflammatory.

Unlike its parent fatty acids, hydroxy fatty acid derivatives are relatively miscible with alcohol and water; in fact, hydroxy fatty acids actually take up water and bond with it. Thus, they "hold" water in the skin and prevent it from evaporating.

This property enables HDA to blend with and fortify the skin's natural hydroxy fatty acids.

Since HDA is a monohydroxy fatty acid similar to those our skin synthesizes, it has anti-inflammatory properties. It's thought that HDA acts in concert with the proteins, carotenoids, and flavonoids in royal jelly to provide anti-inflammatory and antiallergenic effects. These effects can occur with either topical application or ingestion.

Royal jelly fed to mice was recently shown to suppress the development of atopic dermatitis-like skin lesions. The mice used for the experiment were specially bred nude mice with immune defects that allowed them to easily develop allergic skin conditions. When an irritating chemical was put on their skin to cause dermatitis, royal jelly provided the animals relief even though it had been ingested rather than topically applied.

How Does Royal Jelly Work Medicinally?

There are six major reasons for the preventive and healing properties of royal jelly. We have already discussed the unique skin healing aspects above.

1. The many nutrients, HDA, antimicrobial proteins, enzymes, and gamma globulin in royal jelly all play a role in its ability to prevent infections and stimulate healthy immune responses.

2. Of these substances, HDA also has an antibiotic effect. Because the structure of this fatty acid is similar to a detergent, it can disrupt the structure of bacterial cell membranes. Royal jelly contains other short-chain saturated fatty acids, which also possess detergent-like antibacterial, antifungal, and antiviral properties.

3. Improvements in cardiovascular health are largely due to HDA, which I speculate acts

similarly to 13-HODE. 13-HODE is a hydroxy fatty acid derived from linoleic acid that's normally present in artery walls, where it inhibits atherosclerosis and blood clot damage.

4. Additionally, royal jelly contains all the B vitamins. It's rich in hormones, phytosterols (mainly beta-sitosterol) and phospholipids (mainly phosphatidyl choline and acetylcholine). These compounds all help lower cholesterol, and if you ate *enough* royal jelly, might make you feel younger.

5. Constituents in royal jelly known to aid wounds, dyspepsia, and stomach and duodenal ulcers include pantothenic acid, phytosterols, certain flavonoids, short-chain fatty acids, and in some cases enzymes.

6. Peptides from digested royal jelly lower blood pressure. It is thought that the enzymes in fresh royal jelly may act synergistically with the peptides.

How to Purchase and Use Royal Jelly

The highest quality royal jelly products usually come from manufacturers with a full line of bee products. It takes professional apicultural, processing, and distribution practices to ensure the integrity of royal jelly because it is exceedingly perishable.

Royal jelly cannot be heated or exposed to light. Fresh royal jelly purchased as a liquid or as soft-gel caps should be stored under refrigeration. There should be an expiration date on the bottle. Don't purchase vials of royal jelly that have been stored at room temperature for an indeterminate period.

A study in Greece found that royal jelly fresh from the hive contained higher levels of enzymes than royal jelly processed for commercial packaging. Imported Chinese royal jelly purchased in a market was even worse—many enzymes measured in the fresh royal jelly were completely absent. Enzymes are degraded in the commercial products by exposure to high temperatures during processing and by prolonged storage at room temperature and under lights. Often poorly marked, undated vials are imported from Asian countries, and there is no manufacturer listed that you can contact if you don't like the product or have questions.

Royal jelly can also be successfully freeze-dried, which keeps it fresh, viable, and stable at room temperature in capsules or tablets. Freeze-dried royal jelly also has the advantage of being concentrated. I personally use freeze-dried royal jelly from a U.S. manufacturer.

Often fresh royal jelly is sold mixed with honey. Honey is a natural preservative for royal jelly, and protects it well if the honey is tightly capped and stored out of direct heat and light. After opening, honey with royal jelly can be stored at room temperature for several months. However, if you don't use it up quickly, or the weather or climate is hot, it's best to refrigerate it after opening.

Doses and Precautions

Always sample a tiny amount of royal jelly when using it the first time. Royal jelly has caused breathing difficulties or asthma attacks in sensitive persons. You can potentially be allergic to specific bee proteins in royal jelly even if you do not react to honey, bee pollen, propolis, or bee stings. Those with severe flower pollen allergies may be allergic to royal jelly since bee pollen is used to make royal jelly.

If you have no adverse reactions, there's no known risk for doses over 10 to 20 grams a day. Always remember that 1 gram of liquid royal jelly is equivalent to 200 to 300 mg freeze-dried—typically the amount in one capsule or tablet.

One to two grams liquid royal jelly is a good daily preventive dose. Use this for improving immunity, fatigue, dry skin, and reducing your risk for colds and flu. If you can afford it, consider doubling your daily preventive dose if you're elderly or immune-suppressed. If you're recovering from serious illness or injury, or intend to use royal jelly to lower cholesterol or blood pressure, or to treat eczema, use 4 to 7 grams liquid royal jelly each day.

Royal jelly works synergistically with other bee products. For example, ulcers and viral infections respond better to a combination of propolis, honey, and royal jelly than they do to any of these products used alone. Royal jelly combined with bee pollen is a highly absorbable natural vitamin supplement. This option is recommended for older or ill individuals who either can't eat much or don't respond to standard supplements.

CONCLUSION

Now you can understand that beehive products are akin to the hundreds of herbal products that we use to improve our health. While born out of folklore and mystery, many medicinal plants have evolved through modern scientific research to become state-of-the-art treatments. Honey is a shining example: consider how quickly it can heal ulcers unresponsive to conventional therapies.

A honeybee colony is an organized society where individual bees have specific roles to protect and maintain the colony. *Bees are phytochemical experts.* They know how to feed the colony properly with honey and pollen. They can protect the hive from disease and invaders by collecting propolis. Bees ensure the colony's survival by making royal jelly from pollen and nectar. Three days of royal jelly consumption protects all larvae from infection and ensures growth. For the queen, a steady diet of royal jelly directly causes extreme growth, sexual maturity, and longevity.

Humans don't have the ability to collect pollen, nectar, and propolis. But we do have the ability to recognize that harvesting is not a quaint insect habit, but rather a sophisticated selection process that we can take advantage of. All over the world, bees find appropriate plants to sustain their hives. Scientists now understand that bees have already done the research and development for us by collecting and concentrating plant materials that provide exceptional nutritional and medicinal benefits.

My family and I have been beehive believers for years. Let me conclude by giving you our favorite uses for honey, propolis, bee pollen, and royal jelly:

- A large jar of raw honey with pollen, propolis, and wax sits on the medicine shelf along with the bandages. We've healed countless cuts, scrapes and burns scar-free. The children enjoy using honey because it never hurts or stings, bandages don't stick to the wound, and they get a little taste of honey to make them feel better.
- You *can* stop a cold in its tracks! When you feel a cold just coming on—quit whatever you are doing—and rest. One day in bed at the onset of a cold will prevent five days in bed later. Take one teaspoon of propolis syrup or two capsules or tablets, 1,500 mg vitamin C, and a dropper of maitake mushroom extract every three hours until you are well.
- It can be hard to get enough fruit, vegetables, and fiber while traveling or working long hours. Try eating one tablespoon of bee pollen and one or two tablespoons of flaxseed meal each day. You will be getting at least half the fiber and produce you need daily with very little time or effort. And these products are easily carried in your luggage, purse, or any other small container.
- Instead of that afternoon coffee "pick-me-up," try royal jelly along with a bee pollen snack bar. Or swirl honey with royal jelly into some plain yogurt or kefir.

Any of these small changes in your life can make a big impact on your health, so why not try something from the hive?

SELECTED REFERENCES

Al-Muffarej SI, El-Sarag MSA. "Effects of royal jelly on the humoral antibody response and blood chemistry of chickens." *Journal of Applied Animal Research* 12 (1997): 41–47.

Al-Waili NS. "An alternative treatment for pityriasis versicolor, tinea cruris, tinea corporis and tinea faciei with topical application of honey, olive oil and beeswax mixture: an open pilot study." *Complementary Therapies in Medicine* 12 (2004): 45–47.

Bell RR, Thornber EJ, et al. "Composition and protein quality of honeybee-collected pollen of *Eucalyptus marginata* and *Eucalyptus calophylla*." *Journal of Nutrition* 113 (1983): 2479–2484.

Bonvehi JS, Jorda RE. "Nutrient composition and microbiological quality of honeybee-collected pollen in Spain." *Journal of Agricultural and Food Chemistry* 45 (1997): 725–732.

Borrelli F, Maffia P, et al. "Phytochemical compounds involved in the anti-inflammatory effect of propolis extract (suppl. 1)." Fitoterapia 73 (2002): S53–S63.

Buck AC, Cox R, et al. "Treatment of outflow tract obstruction due to benign prostatic hyperplasia with the pollen extract Cernilton, a double-blind placebo controlled study." *British Journal of Urology* 66 (1990): 398–404.

Campos MG, Webby RF, et al. "Age-induced diminution of free-radical scavenging capacity in bee pollens and the contribution of constituent flavonoids." *Journal of Agricultural and Food Chemistry* 51 (2003): 742–745.

Ceglecka M, Wojcicki J, et al. "Effect of pollen extracts on prolonged poisoning of rats with organic solvents." *Phytotherapy Research* 5 (1991): 245–249.

Cohen HA, Varsano I, et al. "Effectiveness of an herbal preparation containing echinacea, propolis, and vitamin

C in preventing respiratory tract infections in children: a randomized, double-blind, placebo-controlled, multicenter study." *Archives of Pediatric and Adolescent Medicine* 158 (2004): 217–221.

Dunford CE, Hanano R. "Acceptability to patients of a honey dressing for non-healing venous leg ulcers." *J Wound Care* 13 (2004): 193–197.

Furusawa E, Chou SC, Hirazumi A, Melera A. "Antitumor potential of pollen extract on Lewis lung carcinoma implanted intraperitoneally in syngenic mice." *Phytotherapy Research* 9 (1995): 255–259.

Gheldof N, Wang X-H, Engseth NJ. "Buckwheat honey increases serum antioxidant capacity in humans." *Journal of Agricultural and Food Chemistry* 51 (2003): 1500–1505.

Iannuzzi, J. "Royal jelly: mystery food (parts I–III). *American Bee Journal* 8 (1990): 532–534; 587–589; 659–662.

Inoue S, Koya-Miyata S, et al. "Royal jelly prolongs the life span of C3H/HeJ mice: correlation with reduced DNA damage." *Experimental Gerontology* 38 (2003): 965–969.

Kamakura M, Mitani N, Fukuda T, Fukushima M. "Antifatigue effect of fresh royal jelly in mice." *Journal of Nutrition Science and Vitaminology* (Tokyo) 47 (2001): 394–401.

Kimoto T, Aga M, et al. "Apoptosis of human leukemia cells induced by Artepillin C, an active ingredient of Brazilian propolis." *Anticancer Research* 21 (2001): 221–228.

Koya-Miyata S, Okamoto I, et al. "Identification of a collagen production-promoting factor from an extract of royal jelly and its possible mechanism." *Bioscience, Biotechnology and Biochemistry* 68 (2004): 767–773.

Liao H-F, Chen Y-Y, et al. "Inhibitory effect of caffeic acid phenethyl ester on angiogenesis, tumor invasion, and metastasis." *Journal of Agricultural and Food Chemistry* 51 (2003): 7907–7912.

Liebelt RA, Calcagnetti D. "Effects of a bee pollen diet on the growth of the laboratory rat." *American Bee Journal* (May 1999): 390–395.

Linskens HF, Jorde W. "Pollen as food and medicine—a review." *Economic Botany* 51 (1997): 78–87.

Mahgoub AA, el-Medany AH, Hagar HH, Sabah DM.

"Protective effect of natural honey against acetic acid-induced colitis in rats." *Tropical Gastroenterology* 23 (2002): 82–87.

Martins RS, Pereira ES, Jr. et al. "Effect of commercial ethanol propolis extract on the in vitro growth of Candida albicans collected from HIV-seropositive and HIV-seronegative Brazilian patients with oral candidiasis." *Journal of Oral Science* (2002): 44, 41–48.

Misirlioglu A, Eroglu S, et al. "Use of honey as an adjunct in the healing of split-thickness skin graft donor site." *Dermatological Surgery* 29 (2003): 168–172.

Molan PC. "The antibacterial activity of honey (part 1 and part 2)." *Bee World* 73 (1992): 5–76.

Molan PC. "Why honey is effective as a medicine: its use in modern medicine (part 1)." *Bee World* 80 (1999): 80–92; Part 2. "The scientific explanation of its effects." *Bee World* 82 (2001): 23–40.

Park YK, Fukuda T, et al. "Suppression of dioxin mediated aryl hydrocarbon receptor transformation by ethanolic extracts of propolis." *Bioscience, Biotechnology, Biochemistry* 68 (2004): 935–938.

Santos FA, Bastos EMAF, et al. "Brazilian propolis: physiochemical properties, plant origin and antibacterial activity on periodontopathogens." *Phytotherapy Research* 17 (2003): 285–289.

Subrahmanyam M. "Honey-impregnated gauze versus amniotic membrane in the treatment of burns." *Burns* 20 (1994): 331–333.

Taniguchi Y, Kohno K, et al. "Oral administration of royal jelly inhibits the development of atopic dermatitis-like skin lesions in NC/Nga mice." *International Immunopharmacology* 9 (2003): 1313–1324.

Tokunaga KH, Yoshida C, et al. "Antihypertensive effect of peptides from royal jelly in spontaneously hypertensive rats." *Biological Pharmacology Bulletin* 27 (2004): 189–192.

Vittek J. "Effect of royal jelly on serum lipids in experimental animals and humans with atherosclerosis." *Experientia* 51 (1995): 927–935.

Vynograd N, Vynograd I, Sosnowski Z. "A comparative multi-centre study of the efficacy of propolis, acyclovir and placebo in the treatment of genital herpes (HSV)." *Phytomedicine* 7 (2000): 1–6.

Other Books and Resources

Bee Propolis: Natural Healing from the Hive by James Fearnley (Souvenir Press, 2001).

Bee Well—Bee Wise: With Bee Pollen, Propolis, and Royal Jelly by Bernard Jensen (Bernard Jensen Publisher, 1993).

Health and Healing with Bee Products by C. Leigh Broadhurst (Alive Books, 2002).

Honey: The Gourmet Medicine by Joe Traynor, Mark Goodin, and Daniel Pouesi (Kovak Books, 2002).

The World's Only Perfect Food: The Bee Pollen Bible by Royden Brown (Hohm Press, 1993).

Online Bee Products Research and Resources

Apimondia—International Federation of Beekeeper's Association: www.apimondia.org

Information and updates on the latest bee research worldwide.

National Honey Board: www.nhb.org

Scroll down to "Honey Research Links" for articles on pollination and more.

International Bee Research Association: www.ibra.org.uk

Source of basic bee research on topics related to health and healing. Look for the *Medicine from the Bees* CD-Rom in their online store.

Commercial Sites and Retail Sales

CC Pollen Co. Phoenix, AZ
www.ccpollen.com

A comprehensive source of bee products, including honeys, propolis, bee pollen, and royal jelly products. Features all natural, wild-collected bee pollen from the high-desert plateaus of the U.S. Southwest, CC Pollen's All-Natural Buzz Bars (the leading bee-pollen snack bars on the market), as well as books and basic information on beehive products. For pet bee pollen and related animal products, see their additional site: www.petpower.com.

Beehive Botanicals, Inc., Hayward, WI
www.beehivebotanicals.com

A full-line bee products company, featuring a wide variety of honeys, propolis, bee pollen, and royal jelly products, unique healing balms, beeswax candles, gift packages, skin and hair-care products with ingredients from the hive.

Comvita Ltd. Bay of Plenty, New Zealand
www.comvita.com

Offers manuka honey and propolis from New Zealand's pristine native forests, as well as a full line of propolis products, including elixirs, tablets, toothpaste, mouthwash, throat spray, cold remedies, and propolis-tea tree oil salves.

Honey Locator
www.honeylocator.com

A resource for learning about more than 300 distinct types of honey from various floral sources across the United States.

Winner's Bee Pollen, Inc., Phoenix, AZ
www.winnersbeepollen.com

Specializes in bee pollen for horses.

GreatLife Magazine

Consumer magazine with articles on vitamins, minerals, herbs, and foods.

Available for free at many health and natural food stores.

Let's Live Magazine

Consumer magazine with emphasis on the health benefits of vitamins, minerals, and herbs.

Customer service:
1-800-676-4333
P.O. Box 74908
Los Angeles, CA 90004

Subscriptions: 12 issues per year, $19.95 in the U.S.; $31.95 outside the U.S.

Physical Magazine

Magazine oriented to body builders and other serious athletes.

Customer service:
1-800-676-4333
P.O. Box 74908
Los Angeles, CA 90004

Subscriptions: 12 issues per year, $19.95 in the U.S.; $31.95 outside the U.S.

The Nutrition Reporter™ newsletter

Monthly newsletter that summarizes recent medical research on vitamins, minerals, and herbs.

Customer service:
P.O. Box 30246
Tucson, AZ 85751-0246
e-mail: jack@thenutritionreporter.com
www.nutritionreporter.com

Subscriptions: $26 per year (12 issues) in the U.S.; $32 U.S. or $48 CNC for Canada; $38 for other countries

INDEX

www.ingramcontent.com/pod-product-compliance
Lightning Source LLC
Jackson TN
JSHW011406130125
77033JS00023B/866
* 9 7 8 1 5 9 1 2 0 1 6 3 2 *